We Shared The
Time Of Her Life

By Anna Lynn

DEDICATION

This book is dedicated to those who are hurting and feel that no one understands their pain. May you come to discover hope and new courage to deal with the heartaches you face, knowing you are not alone in your thoughts and struggles. May you emerge from your suffering to live life to the fullest. May you trust God to work out His best plan.

CONTENTS

Acknowledgments

Introduction

Chapter 1   Interrupted by Friendship

Chapter 2   The Lake House Vacation

Chapter 3   Heart to Heart

Chapter 4   Common Ground

Chapter 5   The Retreat

Chapter 6   Cut Me Some Slack

Chapter 7   Overcoming Barriers

Chapter 8   Prayer for Strength

Chapter 9   The Ultimate Adventure

Chapter 10   Providential Meeting

Chapter 11   Looking Back

Chapter 12   Coping

Chapter 13   Three Kinds of Love

Chapter 14   An Epilogue

What Is Your Story?

ACKNOWLEDGMENTS

The production of this book has been long and heart wrenching. I will forever be grateful to those who encouraged me to keep at it.

Thank you most of all to my husband, who never complained about my late (or early) hours of writing and dominating the computer. You believed in me before I had written the first page. You have continued to believe in me and praise my work through many formats and hundreds of revisions. When I put it on the shelf and said I couldn't do it, you inspired me to keep going and told me it was great, even when it wasn't. Thank you for challenging me to share the story we both believe deserves to be told.

Thank you to those who reviewed my manuscript, gave me feedback, and helped make this a better book: Gene and June, Millie, Worth, Sam and Dee, Karen, Bea, Ted and Pat, Fred and Susette. Your insights were invaluable. You each contributed in immeasurable, countless ways. Bless you.

Thank you, Michelle *(MMG Photography, 5671 E. McMullen Road, Floral City, Florida 34436)* for your fabulous picture. You have a great talent for capturing beauty.

And, finally, thank you to Mark for sharing the time of Jennifer's life with us. Thank you for agreeing to let me express her story without camouflaging your failures. Your transparency is penetrating as you provide an honest, behind-closed-doors look at life in the home of someone terminally ill. I believe your perspective is a powerful aspect of the book.

INTRODUCTION

Moments come and go. Some pass quickly as they slip unnoticed into obscurity. Others linger as though their lifespan is not exhausted.

The scenes behind me have been replaced by another landscape, but every so often I go to the door of yesterday and gently open it. I peer into memories that still remain vital and alive. They call to me because they refuse to be ignored. I am refreshed as I absorb, once again, the lessons I was taught during a challenging, yet wonderful chapter in my life. I have found healing for my bruised emotions as I relive that brief arrest of time that is desperate to be claimed and not forgotten. Though this time period made me dig deeper for God's strength than I'd ever had to dig before, the rewards of God's grace were compounded.

I will leave ajar, ever so slightly, the door to my memories so we both can pass through and capture the glimmer of life that still remains there. I invite you to renew your courage as we walk together to find hope for the challenges of our lives. May you discover the principles found beneath the surface and look at them in the light of your own story. May you benefit from knowing our failures, as well as our successes.

I find myself inadequate to accurately define the dynamics of my experience, but as I stand in its shadow, I am humbled to begin the story and let you overhear the conversation of a short, but poignant shared moment with Jennifer. It is a true story, although I've changed the names and most places to protect the privacy of her family.

As you walk with me down the avenue of days gone by, may you benefit from meeting Jennifer. She was ordinary, yet unique. She was fun and she was faith strong. She was real. She was awesome.

Anna Lynn

"What is a friend? I will tell you. It is a person with whom you dare to be yourself." - Frank Crane

She was a mom, a pediatric nurse, a preacher's wife. Her sense of humor often amazed me as it emerged in unexpected ways. She generated enthusiasm and appreciation for the simple things in life. She had breast cancer and her doctor blindly considered her a survivor.

I learned much from Jennifer: how to hang a spoon on my nose; how to delicately say what I mean without throwing a fit; and how to rise above difficult circumstances when the odds are stacked against me. I haven't perfected all these lessons, especially the spoon.

I met her when my husband, Rich, and I attended a conference held at Jennifer's church. She and her husband, Mark, soon became our dearest friends. It felt as though our lives had been interrupted by this compelling friendship. It had been searching for us and we came together to share an interlude of time. Our relationship was a riveting force that penetrated our spirits. It immersed us in more wholeness than we'd ever known. In terms of longevity it was brief, but in terms of impact, it was forever. This is Jennifer's story.

I noticed her across the room the day we met. She was shorter than I, a bit rounded from childbearing yet very attractive. Her champagne-blonde hair was well styled and casual which accentuated her pretty face. She carried herself with grace and barely showed signs of aging. She made her way across the room and extended her hand to shake ours.

"Welcome to California," she began. "How was your trip?"

"It was long," I responded. "Good, but sorta long. I'm just thankful to be here to enjoy your sunshine. It made the whole trip worthwhile!"

After contrasting our weather back home to California's and exchanging small talk Jennifer told us that the conference had arranged housing for all the guests. "You and Rich will be staying with Mark and me," she explained.

That was the one element of the conference that we didn't like and nearly didn't attend because of it. We didn't want to stay in the home of strangers, but that attitude quickly changed after meeting Jennifer. I had noticed right off that she was articulate, well groomed and didn't drool on her shirt, so I relaxed and got excited about getting to know our hosts.

Jennifer's laughter was infectious. I immediately felt comfortable, as though we were good friends already and could see into each other's souls. One late evening as our husbands talked in another part of her home, Jennifer shared with me the story of her skirmish with breast cancer three years prior. A mastectomy had immediately followed diagnosis, whereupon she began chemotherapy. Following treatment she regained her energy, continued to work, and turned her focus away from cancer. I had a lot of questions about that period of time in her life and her responses revealed a lady of great faith and depth. I was in awe of her spiritual strength. Our hearts embraced as we discussed the many issues that can arise during times like that. Once past the initial discussions about breast cancer, the topic rarely came up again.

A little over two years later Mark accepted a job 50 miles from our home. We were excited at the prospect of our friends moving closer to us. Our relationship would no longer be confined to long-distance phone calls and occasional visits. We decided to plan an "adventure" a month. We'd sit and dream up fun things to do that we'd all enjoy. Some adventures were elaborate, while some were very simple. At times the list of ideas grew long, as well as

7

ridiculous and amusing. On one occasion, Mark launched into a detailed description of the perfect adventure.

"I have this **great** idea," he began, nearly growling the word **great** like Tony the Tiger. His smile was big and his eyes grew wide with excitement. He leaned forward on the edge of his chair and waved his arms as he continued. "We can inner tube across Lake Michigan!"

Jennifer and I looked at each other in disbelief. Speaking simultaneously we chanted, "Inner tube across Lake Michigan??!!!"

"Yes, yes," he continued, his words coming faster. "It could be a super adventure!"

"Are you crazy?" I retorted. "Do you know how **big** Lake Michigan is?"

"Well, yes, I guess it's kind of big I suppose, but we could do it!" His excitement mounted as he went on. "We would all enter into a couple months of physical training to get us in shape. We could go to the gym a few days a week. We could all fit that in couldn't we? Then we would meet on the weekends and jog together."

"Jog?" Jennifer quickly interjected. "Jog?!!"

"Sure. We could jog. It'd really get us in shape fast – and lift weights. We could lift weights!" His vision was increasing in momentum. His arms continued to thrash and his smile further increased, proportionate in size to the fervor of his sales pitch.

My pessimistic wet-blanket side kicked in as I asked, "What if we fall out of our inner tube or what if a storm hits when we're in the middle of the lake?"

"Well, we'd have people in boats that would escort us," he grinned, certain he had all the bases covered and could convince us. "They'd follow us to be sure we were safe and give us drinks and food. It'd be perfect. We might even be on television!"

"We'd be on television all right!" Jennifer laughed. "They'd show us on the 6 o'clock news as the rescuers pulled our lifeless bodies from the bottom of the lake!"

Mark ignored my giggle while Rich sat quietly with a faint smirk on his face. He in no way intended to enter the conversation. He knew he was not going to have to sit in an inner tube, and was confident Jennifer and I would shoot the necessary holes in this proposed adventure enough to kill it. He calmly let us do the dirty work.

Mark got an A for effort in giving his dynamic presentation, but try as he might, he was unsuccessful in getting our endorsement to forge Lake Michigan. He slumped back in his chair sighing as he faked a deflated ego and finally compromised with activities that felt more appropriate for this 40-something group.

One September weekend our chosen adventure was a hike in the mountains. It was a cool fall day, perfect for hiking. We headed out early Saturday morning with backpacks loaded with granola bars, sandwiches and drinks. We were excited about spending the day together and our enthusiasm about our adventure mounted. After pulling into the parking lot at the trailhead, Rich showed Mark his 22 caliber handgun. In typical Barney Fife fashion he squatted slightly and shoved his artillery into its holster.

"The bears and mountain lions better keep their distance if they know what's good for them!" he boasted. "My aim is deadly!"

"Well, I feel safer already knowing you're going to protect us from bears and mountain lions with that 22," I responded. "How many bullets did Andy let you have today?"

Hardly a serious word was spoken as we followed the winding trails. The sun shone brightly through the trees as we made our way along the mountainside. A couple miles into the hike, though, Jennifer needed to stop to catch her breath. She pulled out an inhaler and breathed the spray deeply into her lungs.

"I think I have some allergies and sometimes this helps me breathe easier," she responded to my look of surprise.

She has allergies? That's the first I'd heard that or seen any indication of it. Why hadn't she said something? I was

9

confused and felt bad that it was hard for her. I wondered why she had let us plan a whole day centered on activity that would impact her like this.

The ascents on the hills were tough, but she was determined to push on, not completely sharing with us the extreme difficulty she was having. As I walked almost every day and she didn't, I considered some of her fatigue natural. She pressed on, but the last stretch back to the car was slow. The two of us hung back while the guys went on ahead. We took our time, taking advantage of the opportunity for girl talk. After completing our hike she was exhausted. But, sadly, we all dismissed it as she slumped into the back of the car and laid her head into the seat.

Our next adventure planned for October was to be horseback riding to view the fall foliage. The trees were beginning to change from green to a spectacular array of gold, orange and flaming red. As their colors usually peak in our area around the second week in October, it seemed the perfect time to go horseback riding through the woods. Just before the scheduled adventure Jennifer had pneumonia. We stopped in to check on her and found her in a contemplative mood. She was more serious than usual as she described to me how she had been feeling.

"I was kind of scared," she expressed. "I thought maybe the cancer had returned."

"Really," I responded. I listened intently as she continued.

Her expressions were deliberate as she began to unfold her thoughts. Her eyes were dark as she sat curled up on the couch. She wasn't a hundred percent yet and it showed. I was a bit surprised when she expressed her fear of cancer. She hadn't shown it, nor had she ever talked to me like that before, not even in times when we were alone away from the guys.

"The last x-rays were clear though, showing only minimal evidence of the pneumonia," she went on. She seemed relieved and we all again dismissed the cough that seemed to linger.

The following February we met midway of our homes for a Sunday afternoon pizza. We talked about the Valentine's Day retreat we were planning to attend the next weekend with friends from their church. As Mark was in charge of the retreat, he asked me if I would incorporate into the program one of the activities I had done at work. As a Corporate Trainer I continually looked for activities that were fun and reinforced my topics and I thought of one that would be appropriate for the group.

As we ate our pizza, Jennifer casually mentioned to me that she was going to have some tests done the following Wednesday. I quizzed her about it but she was vague and so nonchalant that I didn't pursue my questions nor become alarmed.

On Friday night we met Mark and Jennifer and the group from their church at a lodge in the remote hills of New York State. There was a lot of activity with assigning couples to cabins and getting them settled. Jennifer seemed unusually quiet and withdrawn. She was evasive when I asked about her tests on Wednesday, so I didn't push the issue. I sensed, though, that something was wrong.

As I talked with Mark just prior to doing my presentation for the retreat, I asked him about Jennifer's tests on Wednesday. He paused, began to say something, and then paused again. His eyes darted away from mine and looked searchingly about the room as though in pursuit of the nearest exit. Couples bustled around us as they prepared for the evening's activities.

"Is everything alright?" I asked.

"Uh, well, uh . . . . . uh, not exactly," he hesitated again.

I was beginning to be alarmed by Jennifer and Mark's evasiveness and I was starting to panic.

"What's going on? What's wrong?" I firmly but quietly pressed him.

"Uh . . . well . . . I'm not supposed to tell you yet," was his almost inaudible response.

"What do you mean you're not supposed to tell me yet?" I whispered. "You have to tell me! You can't let me wonder like this. Tell me what's happened. What did she find out?" I demanded.

I watched intently as he struggled to find his words. The room around us was filled with laughing couples bent on making the most of this getaway. Jennifer was a short distance away talking with one of the women. Their faces and voices seemed to fade into the distance as he quietly responded.

"She didn't just have tests on Wednesday. She actually had outpatient surgery to have a lump removed from her remaining breast and another from her neck. Uh . . . . both were malignant. But she didn't want you to know yet. She didn't want that to be the focus of the weekend. She wants this weekend to be fun and didn't want it to detract from anything. Please don't tell her I've told you. Please don't say anything," he pleaded.

I immediately went limp as his words hit me with the force of a sledgehammer. The news kept resounding through my brain as I went into shock and began an internal process of grieving.

"I won't say anything," I responded. "Thank you for telling me."

I continued to prepare for my part in the retreat and when it was over, numbly found a chair to ease the deep ache in my stomach that wouldn't go away.

"It's back," I silently repeated over and over to myself. "It really is back."

I went on in a rather out-of-body type way, pretending everything was fine. I let Jennifer have her space, smiling and talking with her as though everything was great. We were both playing a game that I hated. What I really wanted to do was hug her and cry. But I wouldn't violate Mark's confidence, nor invade her privacy. I'd wait until she chose the time to talk. The evening dragged on as I made small talk with couples I didn't know and counted the hours to when I could be alone with my husband and release my emotion.

Jennifer participated in all the activities that weekend. On Saturday afternoon she joined a small group of us that decided to go horseback riding. It was snowing and the wind was chilling. The thermometer didn't rise above 20 degrees all day. As I shivered in the saddle atop my horse, I grumbled about the cold and buried my face in a scarf tied around my neck. Jennifer rode silently behind me and didn't offer a word of complaint.

"How can she do this?" I thought to myself.

Two years earlier I'd had breast surgery and I remembered how I felt afterwards. I knew some of the physical discomfort Jennifer was experiencing. What I couldn't begin to imagine, though, was the emotional pain she was going through. Her fortitude on that cold Saturday afternoon was only the beginning of the unique demonstration of grace and determination I was to witness in my friend.

The mood the next day was solemn as Mark gathered the four of us together in the lodge during a lull in the retreat activities. Jennifer was ready to talk. She was firm as she responded to the tone of the moment, "Look, I don't want cancer to become my identity. I want to just continue doing all the things we have been doing together and go on. I want us to meet for pizza and have our adventures and live our lives like we have been up 'til now."

Her exhortation was strong and deliberate. "I don't want this to become my identity" she reemphasized. "I want to live my life apart from cancer. I don't want who I really am to be lost because of an illness. I don't want people to see a patient so wrapped up in herself and her treatment that they don't see the real me. I want to fully live. Please help me do that."

Jennifer rarely used the word cancer after that day. In reference she spoke only of "the disease" as though the word itself was poison and she refused to let it pass over her lips. She wouldn't lend dignity to the devastating term.

Within a short period of time Jennifer underwent a series of tests to determine if there were further sites of concern.

I'll always remember the Wednesday evening call around 9:00 p.m. I was pleased to hear her voice.

"Hi! How are you doing?" she cheerfully asked.

"I'm doing good," I responded. "How are you doing? Have you found out anything yet?"

She spoke with calmness and ease. "Yes, I got the results back. The tests showed that the disease is widespread. The lungs, liver, skull, chest wall, kidneys, breast, neck, and probably any place else I hurt . . . ." she went on describing the extensiveness of her condition.

I felt weak. It was as though I was watching this episode as a bystander, not a participant in the scene. I flinched at each word. The tone of her voice was cheerful yet matter of fact.

"They told me there is no cure. I can undergo treatment that might buy me some time. I could have chemotherapy, radiation, a bone marrow transplant, but that would only give me a little more time. The outcome will still be the same. I know you may not like this, but I've decided not to pursue any type of treatment."

She was a nurse and understood what she was dealing with by refusing treatment. I couldn't comment on her well thought-through decision. I don't remember my words exactly, only my grief and struggle to know what to say. "I'm sorry. I'm so sorry," I choked.

"I'm really okay," she said in an attempt to comfort me. "I have an incredible peace. It's not an act either. I'm not trying to pretend to be strong. I don't want to play the hero. This is not an act for anyone. I just feel such peace. Not to say I haven't shed tears. I have. But God has calmed my spirit and I'm doing fine."

After saying our good byes and hanging up, I stoically handed the phone to Rich who was standing nearby listening. He held the phone at his side as he waited for the details. He winced at my words as tears filled his eyes.

"In good times and bad we need friends who will pray for us, listen to us and lend a comforting hand and an understanding ear when needed." - Beverly LaHaye

"What do we want to take to the lake house?" I asked. "Is there anything other than our clothes and food that we'll need?"

"No, the house is completely furnished," Jennifer replied. "It has everything that we'll want. I can't wait until we get there! This winter was just too long and snowy. A week at the lake is just what I need!"

Jennifer and I had shared many outings together with our husbands, but this was our first real vacation alone to relax and spend time together. We were about to begin a vacation that peaked on the timeline of my life. The plan was not complicated. We were going to her sister's lake house to spend a week relaxing and soaking up some sun.

The air was warm and the sun bright as I headed up the interstate to pick up Jennifer. After an hour's drive I pulled into her driveway and noticed her outline in the dining room window. Her hair fell down across her face as she leaned forward to wave. Before I was out of the car she bounced energetically toward me with her purse over her shoulder and car keys in her hand.

We greeted with a hug, after which she said, "I'll drive. I've got everything loaded into my car. All we need to do is put your things in and we can go."

"What do you mean, put my things in?" I quizzed. "I thought I was driving."

"Yeah, yeah, I know, but I had all this stuff I wanted to take. I woke up early and figured I might just as well get it loaded so we could leave when you got here," she smirked.

"All what stuff?" I returned. "What are you bringing?"

With my hands planted firmly on my hips in playful disapproval, I walked to her car and looked into the back seat.

"What is all this?" I muttered. "Look at all the food. You know, I brought food, too! Looks like we could feed the whole neighborhood for a month with the food we've got! And four books? How many books can you read in a week? And what's this? The drawer to your kitchen table! Why did you bring the drawer to your kitchen table?"

"Well, I'm refinishing my table and thought maybe I'd get a chance to spend some time this week working on the drawer," she smiled.

"You are unbelievable," I retorted. "Okay, so we can start a food bank, refinish furniture, read four books, sun bathe, go swimming and . . . . Oh, my!" I spouted off. "You are such an overachiever!" I laughed, shaking my head. "How long did it take you to pack everything? What time did you get up?! You are so crazy!"

Jennifer just laughed at my exaggerated rebuke. I smiled in amazement at her determination as I unloaded my car.

Jennifer slid behind the wheel as I crawled into the passenger seat. Time became a nonentity as we headed up the highway together. We laughed and chatted incessantly to catch up on the latest details of our lives.

"Doesn't it feel good not to have any responsibilities for an entire week?" Jennifer asked.

"Unbelieveable," I sighed. "We do have one responsibility though."

"No . . . . really? What's that," she returned.

"Well, we do have to figure out when we're gonna eat all this food," I grinned.

The drive to the lake house seemed brief as we absorbed ourselves in conversation. Jennifer was full of energy and her laughter filled our discussion.

There was an essence of excitement in the air, mingled lightly with a shadow of sadness. The sun's rays bounced through the windshield and highlighted the deep shade of yellow in Jennifer's eyes, a stark reminder of her illness. I noticed that the remaining evidence of jaundice was slightly camouflaged by her sun-tanned skin. Cancer was leaving its mark on the body of this vivacious young woman, my dearest friend.

As we pulled into the driveway of the lake house I admired the neatly kept home with the backdrop of the lake. Summer flowers and large trees accented the well-groomed lawn.

Jennifer and I climbed out of the car, grabbed a couple of our bags and headed up the walkway to the front door. During the grand tour of the house Jennifer told me that the largest bedroom overlooking the lake was mine.

"This is beautiful, Jennifer," I responded. "I love how the house is decorated and the view of the lake is wonderful. Can we just spend the summer here?" I laughed.

I worked to quickly get us settled by emptying the car and unpacking the boxes and bags. After everything was in place, we retrieved lawn chairs from a storage shed at the side of the house and carried them lakeside and relaxed.

"I love this place," Jennifer sighed as she leaned back into her chair. "It's a great place to unwind and think deep thoughts."

"You are so right," I agreed. "This is excellent. Thanks for asking me to come here with you, even if you wouldn't let me drive!"

Suddenly I remembered the camera. I wanted to be sure to capture all the elements of our vacation together so I ran to my room to retrieve it.

"What are we going to set it on?" I wondered as we glanced around the yard.

"How about that table over there," she replied.

Jennifer posed in her chair while I set up the camera. The flag over Jennifer's right shoulder waved gently in the breeze. The blue from the sky and lake blended in harmony. The trees shaded part of the lawn from the sun. This would be a perfect picture. I started the timer on the automatic setting and headed for my empty chair by hers as Jennifer began to laugh.

"Run, Forrest, run!" she taunted. "You can do it!"

My legs flailed recklessly; my rhythm seemed about half a beat off. I felt awkward and silly. Jennifer's snickering was contagious and I panted and snorted my way across the grass. I spun and quickly aimed my backside at the empty chair by hers. I was settling, almost down, when the camera mocked my efforts with a jeering click. Our laughter mounted, then subsided, only to erupt again. We felt like two schoolgirls on the playground during recess. The pressures and realities of life had diminished and we felt the freedom of youth. The harsh truth of illness was denied and we embraced life in its simplest and purest form. It wasn't a perfect picture, but it was a perfect day.

Morning blended into afternoon while the horizon fused with gathering clouds. A slight breeze dimpled the surface of the water and the sky began to darken.

"I'm getting hungry. How about you?" I asked Jennifer.

"I think I am, too. It's been a while since I ate breakfast. Let's just get something quick and keep it simple," she responded.

We headed for the kitchen and assessed our stockpile of food. "How about sandwiches?" Jennifer suggested.

"Sounds good," I replied and began to pull things out of the refrigerator and start the sandwiches and a salad while Jennifer walked out onto the sun porch. I wasn't sure what she was doing but suddenly the wind accelerated and the force of the air through the open kitchen window slammed the door shut behind her.

I noticed raindrops began to prick the lake's surface. Within seconds the splatter against the water increased as the drops grew thick. Heavy beads of water began to blow through the open kitchen window and I rushed to close it. The loud torrent beat fiercely against the panes of glass. Blankets of rain began to hammer the side of the house.

Suddenly the sun porch door opened and I heard Jennifer's faint holler, "Anna, help me!"

At the doorway I saw the rain, driven by a gale-like wind, shooting horizontally into the room. Jennifer

18

struggled frantically to close windows. I hadn't realized it, but while I was unpacking the car, she had opened all the large windows on the porch. I bolted through the door. Uncertain of the mechanics securing each one, I began pulling and tugging at the windows.

"How do these releases work?" I shouted over the noise of the wind, half gargling my words as the rain blasted me in the face. She responded, but I couldn't understand what she was saying. I yanked on the windows and we somehow got the last one shut. We stood face to face in disbelief.

"Can you believe this?!!" Jennifer groaned, still in shock. Water was everywhere.

"Everything is SOAKED!!!" I whimpered.

We swayed, cold and shivering, laughing at the dripping image of each other.

"We are so wet!" Jennifer squealed. Our clothes clung to our bodies as our hair streaked onto our faces. Trying to dry our faces with wet hands smeared mascara down our cheeks.

"You look like a drowned raccoon," I muttered through my laughter.

The water sloshed under her sandals as Jennifer deliberately splashed me.

"Look at your hair!" Jennifer giggled.

"Who in the world opened all these crazy windows?" I said.

"I don't know," she returned. "I don't know, I don't know" she kept mumbling as we paced back and forth laughing.

"How are we ever going to get this dry?" I asked. "Your sister is going to kill us!

"Yeah, I think you're right! We are in big trouble!"

We quickly began sopping up the water on the porch. Our work was often interrupted by pointed comments about the other's appearance. We did look pretty pathetic, but we didn't care. We just had fun.

Once done, we changed into dry clothes and returned our thoughts to lunch. The bread on our sandwiches had dried out, but we were hungry enough that it didn't matter. We settled in around the table thankful to be finished with the cleanup.

The rain and wind continued to blast against the house. Jennifer's blonde sun-streaked hair framed her fragile face and appeared as though it was untouched by our watery predicament. Mine, on the other hand, hung half-heartedly, obvious evidence of our fight against nature. It seemed in a way almost symbolic of how Jennifer was able to deal with the difficulties of life that had drenched her. She handled them well and appeared practically untouched.

As we sat at the table following lunch Jennifer began to cough. The exertion of the day, along with talking so much, had taken its toll. Her cancer-weakened body could withstand only limited activity. Her cough became incessant and would cause her to vomit if she couldn't regain control. Knowing the consequences, I encouraged her to go rest, which she resolutely did.

I cleared the dishes, cleaned up the kitchen and fixed a cup of coffee. I grabbed a book and sank into the large overstuffed chair in front of the stone fireplace. As I sipped my coffee I eyed the tall oil lamps on either side of the mantle. I wondered if we might need to use them if the storm took out the electricity. A large wood captain's wheel hanging above the lamps seemed to tremble as the forceful wind continued to batter the house. The trees along the driveway tossed small branches to the ground. The storage shed door blew open and smacked against the side of the house. It continued to bump and thud.

I could hear Jennifer cough in the bedroom behind me. I prayed hard and sympathetically for God to enable her to rest. I prayed more intensely and longer that He would miraculously heal her.

As I listened to the storm I began to reflect back on what Jennifer told me shortly after her diagnosis. She had begun slowly, and her words troubled me.

"After I regained my strength following chemo treatments from my first cancer I felt really good. I went back to work and things were going well for me. I did fine for a long time – over five years. You know how good I was doing. I was fairly confident that the cancer would not return. I mean, you can't dwell on that for the rest of your life. I wasn't a pessimist. I lived my life thankful to be healthy and able to do the things I wanted to do. I enjoyed life. I didn't live in fear nor imagine that every little ache or pain was the return of cancer."

"Yet when I began feeling very tired all the time, beyond the normal fatigue I felt at the end of a day, it began to concern me. I didn't say anything to anyone. I just made an appointment to talk with my doctor. But he didn't take me very seriously. He treated me like I was a wimpy, whiny hypochondriac and suggested that my symptoms were all in my head. He said that I had passed my five-year mark and I should stop worrying about cancer. So I did. He made me doubt what my body was telling me."

I was angered. I could not believe that her doctor lightly dismissed her complaints. Why didn't he follow through with tests that could have spotted trouble? His neglect plunged her through a crack in the medical profession that should never exist.

How do you spot that one doctor among hundreds who has grown complacent and arrogant enough to dismiss symptoms he should investigate? At what point do we ignore our trust in him and seek other counsel? How do we legitimize our feelings and draw the line between paranoia and pushing the envelope? I must have asked those questions a hundred times, but no one asked them with more intensity than Jennifer. After all, she was a nurse. She wished she had researched her needs for herself. She regretted letting her trust of this doctor corrode her better judgment. She wished she had followed through with what her body was telling her. She was suffering the consequences of not being more aggressive and insisting on proactive measures that could have assured her continued health.

She told me after learning of her condition that the pediatrician she worked for said, "Well, I guess I'm not completely surprised about the cancer, what with the cough you seemed to have and all."

I wished he had nudged her to have some testing done. Why didn't I encourage her when I heard her cough? The word "why" is so small yet insidious, and it plagued my waking hours and haunted my sleep at night.

CHAPTER 3   HEART TO HEART

"A friend is one to whom one may pour out all the contents of one's heart, chaff and grain together, knowing that gentle hands will take and sift it, keep what is worth keeping and with a breath of kindness, blow the rest away." *- George Eliot*

The storm continued but Jennifer's coughing ended. I listened to the wind whip sheets of water against the windows. I was thankful Jennifer was able to sleep through the turmoil that was raging, both outside the lake house and within her body. She struggled so to be whole while living in her weakened body. I refilled my coffee cup and let the words on the pages of my book fill my mind. After a couple hours I heard movement in Jennifer's room.

Approaching behind me she said, "Hi, whatcha reading?" Her greeting was cheerful and her voice strong.

"A book by Chuck Coleson," I responded. "It's good stuff. Did you have a good nap?"

"I really did. Once I stopped coughing I listened to the storm for a couple minutes and then I was out. I feel really good right now!" she said as she settled into the chair across from me. "I feel soooooooooo good!"

The fatigue in Jennifer's face had disappeared and she looked amazingly refreshed.

"That's excellent! You look really good!" I responded. "You slept through a real wild storm. The storage-shed door came open and kept banging against the side of the house and I was afraid it would keep you awake. I thought about going out and closing it, but was afraid I'd get blown clear to Cleveland if I stuck my head out the door. The trees kept whipping like reeds in the sand. I'm thankful one of them didn't come down on the house."

"Well, let's go see if everything's okay outside," Jennifer said as she bounced from her chair. The air was again clear and warm. Small branches and twigs were strewn everywhere. The grill was on its side and a garbage can lid was pressed up against the neighbor's shrubs. The lady next door paced back and forth, her arms planted on her hips as she assessed the damage to her roof.

"What a storm," she sputtered. "A tornado in the next county," she went on fitfully.

Jennifer and I appraised the condition of her sister's lake house as the neighbor trailed off.

"Things look pretty well intact here," we agreed. With everything returned to their proper places, we settled into lawn chairs and viewed the lake that was again smooth like glass.

"Can you believe how still the air is?" Jennifer commented. "What a contrast to earlier."

"Yeah, you know it!" I laughed. "My ears are still ringing from the force of that water hitting me in the face!"

"How abruptly things can change," I reflected to myself, speculating as much about Jennifer as I was the weather. One moment life can be picturesque, the next it can be in turmoil. How quickly our dreams can be hurled to the ground like the small limbs scattered across the yard, the crude rhythms of illness hammering away our strength.

Jennifer smiled as she said, "It's so easy to be here with you. I like the fact that I don't feel like I have to entertain you. I needed to go lie down, yet I knew you'd do your thing and be content."

"Sure, well, just feel free to ignore me any time you'd like," I laughed.

"Seriously," she continued. "I appreciate you making it easy for me to talk about my illness, too."

"I want you to be able to talk about it, Jennifer." I replied. "I need you to talk about it. But sometimes I don't know what to say, or how to say what I really want to express to you. I don't always know if you're comfortable with our talking about your sickness. I don't want to pry or invade territory that is too personal or painful for you. I certainly don't want to pretend to understand what you're going through, because I don't. I don't know. I just care. I want you to say the things that are beating you up inside. I want you to purge and get them out so they don't eat you up. But, sometimes after we've talked a while about how you've been doing, you'll say, 'No more sick talk!' And, that's okay. You should call the shots. Help me to know, though, when we can talk about it without you being uncomfortable."

"You know why I say no more sick talk?" she responded. "Remember the weekend of the retreat at the lodge when I said that I didn't want my illness to become my identity?"

"Sure, I do. I'll never forget that weekend."

"Well, that's why I sometimes say that. It's not that I don't want to talk about it. It's that sometimes we need to move away from it so we can communicate about other things. I don't want my life focus to be my sickness. I need to hear about the things that are happening in your life. I want to share those experiences with you and broaden my own world by joining into the things that are going on with you. It helps me look beyond myself and my own circumstances to share the good things that are happening around me. And when you think about me, I don't want your thoughts to just be about my illness," she continued. "I want you to think about the fun that we have and the neat adventures we share. I think that you need to move away from too much sick talk also because it can become too depressing for you if that's all we dwell on. You are one of my support systems, and you can't help encourage me if you're overly depressed about my situation. We need to have a balance so we can help each other."

"Hummmm. How'd you get so smart?" I asked.

I loved days like this when Jennifer's thoughts flowed easily like fluid from an overturned jar. They'd splash fluently and quickly. I liked to explore the mysteries of life with her and look through the window of her soul and see her heart. I appreciated her sharing her insights because the last thing I wanted was for her to close her spirit to those of us around her who were healthy.

"I want people to be comfortable talking to me about my illness," Jennifer continued. "When they aren't comfortable, I become uncomfortable. But, there's such a fine line in all this. Sometimes people press me for too much information, which makes me want to back away. They need to be there for me but they need to take it slow. I'm sometimes evasive about doctor appointments. I don't like to have people call me the same day they know I've been to the doctor. I realize they are concerned about me, which I appreciate, but when the news is bad, I need time to process it. It may be a day or two – or more – before I'm ready to talk about it. I want to be in control of that type of thing and not be pushed to talk about it before I'm ready. I get tight with information because of my desire to control it. But people don't understand that. I've heard that some think I'm just being too private. They don't think I'm handling it well. What they probably mean is that I'm not handling it like they want me to!"

"Another aspect to this whole thing is that sometimes people have asked me how I'm doing and I respond 'good.' They haven't always understood that when I say I'm doing well, it sometimes can be a self-fulfilling prophecy. Saying I'm doing good helps me to do better. If all I talk about is how bad I feel, I would only continue to feel worse. I'm not trying to be deceptive. I just need to focus on what is positive."

"And, believe it or not, sometimes it even helps me to do better if I don't go to the doctor. Even though my decision was not to have aggressive treatment, the doctor still wanted to see me regularly. But, when I continually saw him, I began to fulfill what he was telling me."

"'One cancer cell divides into two cells, two divide into four as the cancer gradually takes over your body and you get weaker and sicker,' he'd say every time I saw him. I got so tired of hearing that little speech of his I could spit!"

Jennifer raised her hands into the air as she said the word spit and thrust her arms forward in disgust.

"Spit?" I questioned.

"Yes, spit!" she smirked. "You know what I mean. My illness and the multiplication of those cells was his focus and it was becoming mine as well. My life subtly became focused on my illness - going to the doctor's office and waiting for the next symptom to surface. The quality of my life was not helped. Now I only go to the doctor when I need something specific to make things easier for me. I improve when I purpose to have a life apart from the disease. Like I told you, I don't want it to be my identity. Self-fulfilling prophecies are powerful and I'm trying to do what's best for me."

"They are powerful, Jennifer," I returned, "and it sounds like you are doing it right."

"Then there's another side to this whole thing of communicating," Jennifer went on. "Sometimes in the confusion of not knowing the best way to approach me about my illness, some people do nothing. If they don't withdraw from me entirely, they avoid conversation of any nature that's related to my problem. Their communication doesn't go beyond the level of a superficial exchange that holds me at an unbearable distance."

"Everybody's thinking about it, but nobody's talking about it," Jennifer said as she leaned back and stretched her arms above her head. "When I went into remission last winter and visited my family in California, I was excited. I couldn't wait to get there. I looked forward to quality time with my family and friends. I felt the best that I'd felt in two years and I was so thankful to be able to travel. It was a wonderful trip for me, but I had some disappointments too. It was so painful that I couldn't tell you about it then."

"Oh, no," I groaned. "What happened?"

"Well, it began with a visit to see my mother-in-law. One of her neighbors that I knew came over to see me. We shared some small talk for a while. She was pleasant and warm. It was okay. She asked about the kids and then

27

asked how Mark was doing. Then it stopped. No more questions. She never asked me how I was doing. She acted like she didn't even know I had been sick. She totally avoided the whole subject. It felt very awkward."

"Well, I went from there to my parents' house. The whole family was there. When I talked to my brother and my brother-in-law, neither one said anything to me about my condition. It was like it didn't exist," she sighed. "There were others there also and when we began talking about my illness, my father went over and picked up the newspaper and started reading it. We talked for some time but the whole while my father sat behind that paper ignoring our conversation. I wanted him to join in. I wanted him to express his sadness. I wanted him to say, 'I'm sorry you are going through this.' I wanted him to say something, anything that just let me know he cared. But he didn't. He just read his newspaper. He's never talked to me about it. He's never said anything. I wish he would. I know it's hard for him. I just wish he'd talk to me, though." Jennifer lowered her voice and rubbed her forehead. "I wanted him to talk to me."

I was stunned. In my mind's eye I could envision that room filled with so much emotion. I felt like I was there as she described the scene. I wanted to change that image for her. In my imagination I wanted to run over and tear that newspaper from his hands. I wanted to grab his shoulders and shake him.

I wanted to scream at him, "Talk to her! Tell her your heart is shattered into a thousand pieces. Hug her and sob. Don't just sit there pretending nothing is wrong. You may not have many more opportunities to express your love to her. Why don't you talk to her?!!"

It's difficult. I know it is, for I had my own struggles with knowing the right thing to say. There were occasions when I wished I could go back and do it better. I'm sure Jennifer's father felt that same thing. Sometimes the gulf seemed so great that words couldn't bridge it. We wanted to bring comfort, but unthinkingly we brought pain. We wanted to encourage, but unknowingly we discouraged. We wanted to help, yet at times we hindered. We all held our own newspapers.

As hard as it was though, we needed to forge on trying to overlook our own pain and focus on her. She wanted our help, not in some pathetic patronizing manner, but just a simple response to her solitude. It was such an unbearably lonely walk she was taking. Jennifer sensed and understood our difficulty. She shared our compassion, except her compassion was for us. She loved us and looked beyond blunders into the faces of imperfect people who meant well.

"He wasn't reading that paper, Jennifer," I offered. "He heard every word. His grief held him behind the newspaper. His capacity to communicate his pain was seared by the reality of the prognosis. He was paralyzed by his feelings. Holding that newspaper was security for him, for to put it down would be to expose the excruciating horror in his heart over the thought of losing you. He couldn't bear it. It was more than he could handle. He loves you more deeply than you can ever realize."

"I know that's true," she smiled softly. Her face brightened and her countenance completely changed, "I know it's true."

"To affect the quality of the day, that is the highest of arts."
- Henry David Thoreau

"Look at me," Jennifer said, interrupting the thoughts she'd had of her father.

"What do you mean? I am looking at you," I returned.

"No, sit still and lean forward a bit," she insisted. I responded to her request by leaning toward her, totally confused and unaware of what was coming next.

"I can still see it," she laughed.

"You can still see what?" I replied looking puzzled.

"The dent in your head," she grinned.

"What dent?" I laughed.

"The dent in your head from Rich smashing your wheelchair into the steel post at the zoo," she giggled. "It's still there. I can see it!"

"No you can't," I smirked.

"Yes, I can," she continued laughing. "You are scarred for life!"

"You've been in the sun too long!" I protested. "It's a wonder I wasn't maimed for life, really. I should have known better than to put my life into his hands like that. He gets sidetracked way too easily. That was sorta crazy. Tell me, though, do I really have a dent?"

"Absolutely!" Jennifer laughed. "It's huge!"

"I don't think so," I laughed. "You are hallucinating! Anyway, in spite of my dent, that was a fun day, wasn't it. Why didn't you want to use a wheelchair?"

"I don't like using a wheelchair," Jennifer responded. "Maybe it's all about the self-fulfilling prophecy thing, I don't know. I feel sad for people who are in wheelchairs dealing with their suffering every day. I'm thankful I'm not that bad at this point. I can walk. I wasn't that sick yet and

30

I didn't want to play the part of an invalid because I wasn't one."

"That's right. You weren't. But had you walked through the entire zoo you probably would have been sick for days afterwards, wouldn't you?" I cautiously asked.

". . . . . .Yes. . . . . I know you're right and that's why I finally gave in when you said you were going to use a wheelchair too. It did make it a lot easier for me seeing you in your wheelchair alongside me. And it was rather interesting seeing people's reactions to two wheelchair-bound women, wasn't it," she joked. "Especially when the guys would push us up to the restrooms and we'd jump out of the chairs and walk inside."

"Interesting doesn't begin to describe that day," I laughed.

The parking lot had already begun to fill with cars by the time we arrived at the zoo that Labor Day morning to share our September adventure. Moms and dads with strollers, teenagers in love walking hand-in-hand, and grandmas and grandpas all made their way to the ticket booth. I was a little apprehensive as the guys unloaded the wheelchairs from the van. Jennifer's face was subdued, and I sensed that although we were making light of it, it was still very difficult for her to use the wheelchair. I could only imagine how she was feeling. I could only further imagine the increased intensity of what she would have been feeling if I hadn't insisted on joining her in this way.

One of the chairs had been around for a while. It was weather worn and, for whatever reason, was missing the footrests. But its serviceability for us was only to provide a bridge between Jennifer and me, and for that it was perfect. I jumped into the chair and began going through a gyration of positions that could comfortably support my feet without having to hold them straight out mid-air. We were light hearted, yet the reality of why we were doing this was ever present. An underlying sadness hid in the shadows waiting to join us.

Curious empty eyes, showing neither compassion nor sociability, watched us make our way to the entrance in our wheelchairs. I was suddenly uncomfortable, feeling conspicuous much like one who was underdressed for the formal party. I felt each questioning intrusive stare. I pulled my eyes away from the vacant emotion displayed on their faces and felt myself withdraw.

"You don't know me, the real me," I thought. "I'm not a freak – not some sideshow mutation. I'm not on exhibition for you to probe and inspect. You came here to look at the animals, not me. Why are you so rude?"

Thoughts whirled inside my head in response to my feelings. Compassion for Jennifer increased as I watched her respond to interrogating glances. I couldn't measure the intensity of her feelings, but was certain they surpassed mine. It's one thing to be playing the role and quite another to be living it.

As we neared the ticket gate I tried to recollect how I had responded to wheelchair-bound people in the past. I questioned my own behavior and wondered if I had at times, in fact, inflicted my own degree of unintentional pain. I think I fell into the category of those who noticed, looked quickly away, and then politely ignored them so I wouldn't be guilty of staring or calling attention to their disability. The absurdity of this behavior was that they are not the limit of their abilities. They are not a breed of their own. *They are me.* They are me with plans for the day and dreams for the future, with failures and successes and frustrating bad hair days. They are me with gifts and talents, fears and joys. They are me – feeling, needing, caring. *They are me.*

I wanted to explain it to the onlookers. I wanted to explain that I lived just like they did every day. I had a job and kids that I loved. And Jennifer did too, except right now she couldn't work. But there was a time she could. There was a time you couldn't keep her down. Her energy was incredible; her laughter contagious. And the only thing that separated their ability from hers right now was perhaps time and the grace of God.

32

"Recognize her beauty and wit," I wanted to yell. "Don't turn away from those eyes filled with love. Don't gawk and look at her as if she is bizarre, but smile your greeting as you would if you were walking shoulder to shoulder with her."

I was beginning to feel overwhelmed with emotion – too much emotion.

"They don't understand," I thought. "They just don't understand."

I wanted to express my feelings to Rich but, although he was right there not a foot behind me, we couldn't easily communicate. Not only was my back to him, but he stood several feet above me. I twisted and turned my face up to his. He leaned down to respond, but we couldn't easily talk. He was pushing the chair hunched over, and I was twisting and straining as we exchanged quiet words. The contrast between our usual easy interchange and this was incredible. We quickly gave up attempting conversation. I felt isolated and detached. It seemed like a sea of arms and chests surrounded me, apparent signs of life, yet only replicas.

"This is not a good thing," I thought to myself. "I don't like this separation."

Jennifer was the only one with whom I could easily talk. I became immediately thankful for the inspiration to have joined her in this manner. It wasn't a brilliant, or sacrificial decision, just one I thought would make her more comfortable and less resistant to using a chair. Now it felt paramount. I became increasingly aware of how secluded I felt being distanced by the short span of height from those around me. How would she have felt distanced from the three of us in this manner? Would it have been another day where the barriers created by her illness drove her emotionally further from us? Could it have been just one more devastating example of the lonely road she was walking?

At times I felt a bit guilty because our chairs were an inconvenience to those around us. For that I felt like apologizing, but I would not give up my vehicle for maintaining level ground with Jennifer. We were on the same plane, experiencing the same things in the same manner. It was unique for both of us, yet the shared adventure made it less formidable. It's not always easy to maintain commonality with one who is ill and I was thankful for this experience. What would have been a physical and probably emotional separation had she done this alone, became a catalyst that induced fun.

I initiated a new approach to deal with the spectators, one perhaps inspired by cockiness, but nonetheless fascinating. As people stared, I wouldn't look away. I held eye contact and smiled. Some smiled back; some glanced quickly aside in reflex. One man stared so long he finally sheepishly said "hi."

More than just a fun day with friends, this adventure had become a study in human nature. I watched people closely, taking in all the nuances that indicated their ease or discomfort with us. I scrutinized their faces and their curiosities. I blatantly smiled my way through the day in search of compassion and friendly expressions. While many expressed kindness, many others were uncomfortable. Their uneasiness created an empty feeling within me, not for myself but for those who would not walk away from their wheelchairs at the end of the day.

Most people were polite and held doors or moved their children so we could see. Others were carelessly unaware and moved directly in front of us obstructing our view.

"Tell him he's blocking you," I whispered to Jennifer.

"Shhhhh," she responded.

"Tell him to get out of the way," I whispered a little louder.

She gave me her "look" that was generally reserved for her kids when they bordered on embarrassing her in public.

"Bump the back of his legs with your foot rest," I whispered again.

"Stop it," she responded laughing out loud.

"Go ahead. I dare you. You're in a wheel chair. What's he going to do?" I returned snickering.

34

Again I got the "look," although she couldn't do it with a straight face.

"Do it," I said without moving my lips. "I double dog dare you! Do it. Do it!"

At that point I was abruptly pulled backwards.

"We're out of here!" Rich laughed and wheeled me in the opposite direction as though I might actually convince Jennifer to maim the guy in front of her.

As the day progressed, Jennifer and I rode side by side as our husbands maneuvered us about. During one long ascent on a hill via a wooden ramp they were put to the test. They began wheezing and gasping midway to the top. They didn't have quite the same high-spirited enthusiasm as when we had first begun. I could hear them groaning to each other as they plodded along, assessing the distance they still had to go to the crest of the hill. It was work and, for my husband in particular, a demonstration of dedication to Jennifer. I was capable of walking up the elevation, but he continued without hint of me doing that. Once at the top, the guys collapsed onto benches.

We sat for a long time and reflected on our day and the curiosities brought on by our unusual adventure. Jennifer and I joked about being at the mercy of our navigators. Her face was contorted as she began belly laughing so hard she could hardly talk: "Did you see how she bounced when Rich ran her into that pole in the building of aquariums?!"

"Oh, my gosh," I replied. "Could you believe that? I saw the pole coming at me but I couldn't do anything about it with my legs twisted to the side like that. He drives the car the same way. He's always looking at stuff here, there, and everywhere but where he's going," I laughed.

"Well that screaming was pretty embarrassing," Rich said. "I wish you'd be a little more composed in public."

"Yeah, right," I giggled. "I thought I was going down. I was sitting so off balance that grabbing the pole after it whopped me in the head was the only thing that kept me from kissing the floor. It felt like I was doing a May Pole dance. I wasn't sure I'd ever stop spinning! How many rotations did I complete? I'm sure I counted at least 47. I'm still dizzy," I said wiping my forehead with the back of my hand.

"You're dizzy, all right," Rich laughed.

"Did you hear the people gasping?" Mark roared. "Here's this poor, pathetic middle-aged woman in her wheelchair being slammed into a steel post. They didn't know what to think, especially when we started laughing at you. I wish I'd had my video camera. We could've made a fortune on *Funniest Home Videos*. Yep, big money!"

Our laughter turned the day into the only one worth living. We extracted every ounce of unblemished value we could from it.

When it was time to go back down the hill, we chose a paved isolated roadway. The descent was steep and as we approached, Jennifer said, "I think I'll walk to the bottom of the hill rather than use the wheelchair."

In reflection, I wondered if it was more for our safety than it was that she preferred to walk. "You know, Jennifer," I responded, "that's a good idea. Two wheelchair runaways would not be a pretty sight!"

The guys were pleased that we wanted to walk and saw it as an opportunity for a challenge. Their wheelchair race was instantaneously planned. They practiced using the brake a couple times then lined themselves up at the imaginary starting line, making sure they were precisely positioned.

"I can't believe they're doing this." I shook my head in disbelief.

"And I can't believe we're encouraging them," Jennifer laughed. "I hope the First Aid Station isn't too far away."

Because of the missing footrests on my chair, Rich was leaning back with his legs stretched straight forward like long stiff boards. Mark was leaned forward with his hands firmly gripped on the side wheels of his chair. Jennifer gave the signal to begin and the two inexperienced drivers began the pathetic race to the bottom of the hill.

"Look at how those wheels are wobbling!" I shouted.

36

"They're swerving all over the road," Jennifer laughed.

We watched and breathlessly wondered which one was going to wipe out first. The wheelchairs were not meant for speed. As the small front wheels hit crevices in the roadway, they spun and turned the chairs in a new direction. Undaunted, the guys hung on and learned fast. They quickly applied new-found wisdom for steering. But soon it was all over. Ahead by 3 lengths, Mark went wildly out of control.

"He's veering to the side," I yelled.

"Oh man, he's screaming like a girl," Jennifer groaned. "Ouch, he just hit the side of the curb."

Mark flew headlong and nearly launched himself into a lunar orbit. He landed spread eagle in a heap with his face firmly planted in the grass. He moaned as he rolled over onto his back, just in time to see Rich cross the finish line. Battered and deflated by the loss, Mark picked himself up and rubbed at the grass stain on the front of his shirt. He retrieved the chair that was on its side next to the curb. He checked it for damage, wiped a piece of mud off his back and limped his way to Rich to congratulate him on the win. Jennifer and I continued our walk to the bottom of the hill and called an immediate halt to their racing careers.

The cool September day drew to a close as we made our way back to the car. We replayed our activities as we bumped through the parking lot. It had been good. The wheelchairs had become a unique part of the adventure and removed the stigma of illness, enabling us to maintain level ground. As we climbed into the back seats of the van, the guys folded up and loaded the chairs. Looking tired but pleased she said, "Thanks."

"Sure," I responded. "It was fun."

"A woman is like a tea bag – you never know how strong she is until she gets in hot water." - *Eleanor Roosevelt*

"I came here to the lake house by myself once," Jennifer said.

"Really?" I responded. "Your sister wasn't here?"

"No, I was alone," she continued. "I needed to get away and sort things out."

"After the diagnosis?" I asked, although I was sure that was when it would have been.

"Yes. I needed time to gain perspective. I needed private space so I could talk with God and sort out the feelings and frustrations my illness had created. This lake house absorbed a lot of tears as I prayed."

"Tell me about it," I said as I leaned forward and focused on each word she shared.

"Well, my life had changed, and I couldn't function at the energy levels I once had. At times it felt like I was being held at arm's length from the life I had known. My body wouldn't cooperate with me so I could do some of the things that I enjoyed. I felt trapped in a body that was deteriorating, and I was helpless to stop it. Sometimes I would wake up in the morning and have this little ache, and it'd make me wonder if the disease was spreading into a new location. Then I'd think, well maybe I just slept wrong. Then I would question if the new pain was real or if the stress of the illness caused imaginary symptoms to coincide with what the doctor was telling me. My emotions were all over the place. I mourned the loss of the life I once had, and I had to come to terms with this new phase of reality."

"I also grieved for the goals and plans that would never be fulfilled with Mark and the kids. I wondered what the future would bring for my children as they entered the world of adulthood. I think the hardest part for me was dealing with the fact that I wouldn't be sharing that aspect of their lives with them. I wouldn't take part in wedding plans or watch new careers develop. I wouldn't see the faces of their newborns that one day would have called me Grandma. Recognizing and accepting that I wouldn't be sharing all the future milestones of their lives with them was hard. It was very difficult."

"Then, I had to sort out some other disappointments. I had to forgive my doctor. It would have been easy to stay angry with him, but it wouldn't have changed the outcome. It would have only generated hatred and I couldn't afford to use up my energy hating anybody. I had to let it go. I had to forgive him. I tell people that you have to manage your own medical care so you don't slip through the cracks. I found out for myself that doctors aren't 100% mistake free. They sometimes forget to file a result or don't call you about something. They don't mean to. Their motive isn't to do that, but you can certainly fall through the cracks. I had to forgive my doctor for his negligent care."

"I also had to forgive myself for not reacting differently to what he had told me. I could beat myself up for the rest of my life, but it wouldn't change anything. It would only make me feel miserable. It is what it is and I had to learn, with God's help, to deal with it and go on. I had to move away from the place where I was."

"Sometimes I would look at those around me and feel left out, too. Their bodies were strong while mine was weak. I wanted to be able to do what everyone else was doing. At times I felt like I was standing on the outside looking in and I had to deal with that. Occasionally it felt as though my family was pulling away from me, but I recognized that I had to let them participate in things that I couldn't do and not feel sad about it. They couldn't carry my burden long term. They had their functions in life to fulfill. When it felt like they faded in support and compassion for me, I came to realize that they could only live my illness in part and then they had to find their own ways to survive all of this, too."

"Your insight is incredible, Jennifer," I responded.

"Well, it didn't come overnight, but I'm thankful I've been able to work through issues I never thought I'd have to face," she replied. "I had a situation with some of my family members. They were concerned about my decision not to have aggressive medical treatment. They adamantly wanted me to undergo treatment. They were ready to fly me here and fly me there if I would just agree to have treatment. At times they defiantly accused me of giving up. I understood their feelings and I let them verbalize their opinions. A person has to allow family members to express themselves. They have to process it as well; that's all part of it. But in the end, they finally came to realize that it was my decision and I would do what was best for me. My new doctor said my refusing treatment was a very mature decision."

"I spent a lot of time reflecting on spiritual healing also. When I first got my diagnosis I came home and picked up a book to read. I don't remember which one it was so I don't know who to give credit to for the concept. It was almost like the author had a formula. It was simple. Open the Bible, find a scripture that says this or that and you will be healed. So I said to myself, 'You are healed!' Regardless of any symptoms, I felt as strong as I could be right at that moment that I was healed. When the kids came home I told them what the doctor's findings were but said, 'Don't worry because I am healed. Scripture says I am healed.' Now I had read that book in one sitting and the next day I started reading another book. Oh, oh. It had a little different approach. In this one I had to quote scriptures three times a day, like breakfast, lunch and dinner. This was the method that this particular author was advocating. It said that I had to get into the Bible. I couldn't expect to be healed if I wasn't in the Word. I had to do it at least three times a day. There was a whole book of scriptures I was to repeat. So I was thinking, 'Oh, no. Well, I guess I'm not healed.' But I

40

couldn't tell the family yet. That was too big a thing to say the next day – 'scratch the first healing.' So I started taking my "spiritual medicine" – breakfast, lunch and dinner. Then I read another book and another book and another book. They all had some different thing to say about supernatural physical healing. I was like, 'What is this, Lord? What am I supposed to do with all this?'"

"One guy said that you have two options when you break an arm. You can go to the hospital or you can say it is not broken. I thought, 'Okay, if I break my arm I'm just going to say it's not broken?' By this time my faith was feeling pretty small because part of me said, 'If my arm's broken, can I REALLY say it's not?' I'm not sure I could do that. And if I couldn't, was it because I didn't have enough faith?"

"I have personally seen a broken arm healed. Mark saw it as well and so did the other associate pastor. We were in Ft. Lauderdale having Bible School for Haitian children who had come over in boats. It was a big thing in Ft. Lauderdale. There was a lot of immigration that way. Anyway, one of the children had fallen on the playground. I knew a broken arm when I saw it. I was a nurse in a pediatric office for years. I'd seen tons of broken arms. This child had a broken arm. There was no question that it was broken. We were ready to take him to the hospital and were asking where his mother was when all these Haitian women came running out from the kitchen. They started speaking Creole French and laid their hands on him and began praying. Now, I didn't see the arm suddenly go straight. All I knew was, when they took their hands off his arm, it wasn't bent any more. It wasn't hanging down like it had been before they prayed. I believe faith in God's miracles can be greater in some countries where they don't have so many things cluttering up their lives. They have to worry about where their bread is coming from the next day. They're dependent on God for their daily existence while we're worried about what color drapes to buy. I believe we can sometimes clutter our world up and close off God."

"Anyway, I was reading all these books and I kept thinking I had the scoop. Here's what we're doing or not doing right. It was like every other day it would be a new thing – another book for me to read. I finally decided that I could never rely on another man to decide God things for me. I had to search the scriptures and figure it out for myself. Some of the books would say that the Bible says this or that. They would paraphrase it. Then when I looked it up, it didn't seem like that's what it was really saying. So, you can't always take somebody else's word for it. There are plenty of good books out there that help and are good guidance for us, but nothing takes the place of the Word of God. Even if you don't understand it when you first read it, if you stick with it, the Lord will enlighten you as to what it actually does mean."

"Years ago I thought I had an insurance policy from God. After I literally got hit by a bus and spent three weeks in the hospital in ICU, and then got cancer #1, I thought, 'Okay. That's it.' I figured enough bad things had happened to me and I could move on untouched by further problems. But, God doesn't hand out insurance policies and you can't ever think you have it all figured out. I believe that I just need to relax when it comes to supernatural healing. I really believe that God wants me to just focus on Him, not even on faith. I think He wants me to focus on Him and have Him be the center of my world."

"I have spiritually grown so much over the past few months. My dependence on God is greater than it ever has been, yet the peace I feel in my heart is still greater. I recognize and accept that if God doesn't miraculously heal me, my days are short here on earth. But, that's okay because I am confident that this life is not all there is. I look forward to one day having a new body in heaven. I will deeply breathe celestial air and I won't cough any more. I won't have any more pain, and because time as we know it doesn't exist in heaven, my family will join me quickly. I won't be lonely for them there. I'll save a spot for you beside a lake and we'll share an adventure together like we've never known. It'll be wonderful. I look forward to meeting Jesus. He's strengthened me when I didn't think I had any strength left. He's comforted me when I felt I was beyond the point of being comforted. He's given me a vision for a wonderful future beyond what this life has to offer. I'm excited about the new life I will have."

"That's amazing, Jennifer," I responded as tears filled my eyes. "That is so beautiful. I'm excited for you, too, but I really don't want you to leave us."

"I know," she said, "but that's God's decision, not ours."

"Ya know what," she continued. I'm getting hungry. What's on the menu for dinner?"

She didn't say the words 'no more sick talk' this time, but I knew she was ready to move away from the heavy subject for a while. "Well," I began as I wiped the tears from my face, "I brought sauce from home that's got some meatballs, sausage and beef in it that we could have over rigatoni. I brought some garlic bread too. I think there's some salad left over from lunch we could finish. What do you think?"

"Sounds perfect," she said as we headed inside. I began to cook the rigatoni while Jennifer got the dishes and added a couple candles in the center of the table. We ate until we couldn't eat any more, and then leaned back in our chairs to drink our coffee.

"One is taught by experience to put a premium on those few people who can appreciate you for what you are."
- Gail Godwin

The candles on the dinner table grew shorter as we drank our coffee and quietly looked out across the lake. Jennifer's voice, almost in a whisper, broke the silence. "It's so peaceful here. I love it."

"I have to agree with that," I returned. "This is so close to being perfect."

Our conversation again turned serious as we began talking about death in a general way, in a way that most people discuss buying a new car.

"I don't think I'd like a viewing."

"Me either," I replied

"Just the thought of 500 people parading by looking at me lying there bothers me," Jennifer said.

"Boy, I know what you mean," I agreed. "I feel the same way. But, you know, when my mom died, there was something about seeing her at the funeral home that brought healing and closure that I wouldn't have had if I hadn't seen her after the hospital. I needed that time to let go and say my goodbyes."

I thought of her children as I spoke. As hard as it would be for them, I thought they might need the viewing to help them handle Jennifer's death.

"Well, I guess I wouldn't mind just family and close friends. But not everybody," she responded. "Not everybody." Her voice trailed off as she repeated it.

"You know, one of the guys in our church died recently and Mark had to go to the funeral home," she slowly continued. "I really didn't want to go, but Mark had to drive about 20 miles to get there and I thought that maybe I should keep him company. When we got there it really bothered me seeing the man lying in that casket. It was awful. It was very upsetting."

Her eyes had a distant look. I could only imagine the full impact that experience had on her.

"I won't do it again. I'll never do it again," she sighed.

We continued to investigate our options for funerals like we were making a joint venture and then began to get silly in our efforts to move away from the heavy topic.

"Five hundred people?" I questioned. "I'm sure you would have more than 500 people coming to your funeral. I bet with the church and all your family, there'd be a lot more than that. It'd probably be closer to 503 people."

Jennifer's laugh was strong as she replied, "Do you really think so?"

"Oh, sure," I giggled. "At least 503. But I don't think I'd generate that many people at my funeral. Not even close. I'm not sure how many would come for me. Maybe six – my kids, husband and brothers. That would probably be it – six."

"Well, that's certainly depressing," Jennifer chuckled.

"Yes, it is," I responded with a smirk. "That really is depressing, isn't it? I'd just die if only six people came to my funeral."

"You'd just die?" Jennifer laughed, working up a serious belly laugh. "You'd just die?! I don't believe you. You are so blonde! Well, do you know what I want you to do?" Jennifer continued in lighthearted fashion. "When I die I want you to get your camera, set it on automatic, run over and stand there by my casket and take our picture together."

We had always had fun taking our pictures together with the automatic setting on my camera, but the image she drew with her words jarred us. She had meant it to be funny, but it engulfed us both in sadness. Tears filled our eyes as she looked down at the table. The reflection of the flames from the candles softened her face. All I could say was, "Oh, Jen."

We worked to regain our composure and tried again to move away from the topic in a more serious manner.

"Jen," I gently said, "tell me some ways people can help someone who is sick like you. What can we do to make things easier?"

She laughed and tipped her head back.

"Well, I've been going to write a book. The title would be **_Cut Me Some Slack!_** I'd tell about all the things people have done that have bugged me, and then in the last chapter I'd forgive them. I know this has been difficult for people. It's been real hard. But the greatest difficulty is mine, and the greatest amount of slack cutting needs to go to the person dealing with the problem, and that would be me."

She then proceeded to share the content of her book with me. There were issues that hurt Jennifer, things that surprised me as she shared her perspective.

"The first chapter in my book would be about my independence. I suppose I am protective of my independence," she began. "It's hard to give up things that I no longer can do. It feels like part of me is being torn away. It's much like a burglar has invaded my home and taken away my most prized possessions. He's rummaged through everything I have, then taken things I've had since I was a kid – things with meaning and significance. The disease sometimes makes me feel like it is robbing me of myself. So I don't want people taking over areas I can still handle."

"As long as I can walk to the kitchen, I want to do my own cooking. It is my family and I want to provide their meals. It's my role and that role gives me an identity, an identity I want to maintain for as long as I can. At times I feel offended when people offer to provide our meals. I can still cook. There are other members of the family in that house, too. If I die, are these people going to continue bringing them their meals for the rest of their lives? My family needs to learn how to do for themselves. I want to prepare them to survive without me, even if it means eating lousy food while they learn to cook. It is something we need to do together, as a family."

46

Jennifer's thought was reasonable, although not understood by everybody. People wanted to help. They needed to feel they could contribute to a family they knew was hurting. A meal seemed a very practical way to do it. But each casserole that entered that home was a reminder that they were out of sync. Their family life was out of whack, not only temporarily but also probably permanently.

Jennifer and I continued to talk as the sun dropped below the horizon, casting a pink glow across the lake's surface.

"What are some other things that people have done that have bugged you?" I asked. "Tell me about the other chapters in your book."

"Are you sure you really want to know?" she smirked.

"Certainly I do. How many chapters am I in," I laughed.

"All of them," she teased. "All of them!"

"Well, I'll be brave," I replied.

Jennifer leaned forward on her elbows and peeled melted wax from the base of the candlesticks as she continued.

"I guess you should expect people to say some unusual things at times like this. One woman from our church told me 'Your weight loss looks great but it's too bad you had to lose it that way.' If she could have just said that I looked good, I would have felt better. Tacking on the end of her sentence took what might have been a compliment and turned it into an insult. Like, it's too bad you're so pathetic that you didn't have the discipline to diet and take that weight off yourself and it took being ill in order for you to do it and you only look good because you are sick." Jennifer took a deep breath then blew it out emphasizing her long exclamation. "I thought about slapping her, but I was afraid she'd hit me back. She's bigger than I am," Jennifer laughed.

"It's not too late, you know," I responded. "We could double team her like those tag-team wrestlers do. I could sneak up from behind and catch her off guard while you nail her in the face!" I laughed.

"Yeah, I can see it in the headlines now," Jennifer giggled. "Preacher's wife attacks a member of the congregation and lands a flying drop kick in the narthex of the church!"

"Yeah, that probably wouldn't be too good," I laughed, "so, I guess we should wait until she goes into the parking lot."

"You're too anxious!" Jennifer giggled. "It's interesting though, isn't it? I struggled so long with my weight, yet when it came right down to it, it's the one thing I had going for me. If I hadn't been overweight, I probably would have been dead months ago. My being overweight was actually a blessing. How's that for ironic! Who would have thought?"

Jennifer ruefully went on, "Then there was the woman who came to console Mark because he had lost his sex life. She said she knew just what he was going through because she was now divorced and was going through the same thing."

"Are you kidding me?" I asked.

"No, I'm not kidding! Maybe she was looking for some action, I don't know," she laughed. "What she didn't know was that we still had a sex life, but it wasn't really any of her business whether we did or we didn't. My husband didn't need her counseling. That offended me."

"You hear some weird things, and you find yourself surrounded by people with opinions they've never had to exercise. They are strangers to my circumstance. People told me about herbal therapies and the right vitamins to take that would help. Then there was the guy who came to me on an investigative search for the demonic influence in my life. He meant well, but his opinion or theology was not consistent with what was happening with me. One person told me 'I will pray that the devil gets out of you.' I'm sick, not demon possessed! My illness is just more severe than the head cold or flu they had last winter. These people believe one thing about supernatural healing, but they've never had to tap into it and use it. It's never been life or death for them so they get simplistic. They make their claims based on a lot of different factors. I had my own beliefs and opinions on the subject also, but then when I

48

found myself with this terminal illness, I realized I didn't know anything about it (supernatural healing). I hate it when people think they have it all figured out for me. If they were one day faced with what I am, their opinions and advice might change. Reality has a way of testing our opinions, pressing us to the edge of our convictions. That's where the light of authenticity shines. We have to hold on to our ideology or push past our opinions to find the truth. I try to be gracious and understanding, but sometimes I get frustrated with persistent theory and insensitivity." Jennifer leaned back to draw a deep breath.

"What else, Jennifer," I said. "What else has bothered you?"

"Well, I've got a whole chapter in my book about confidentiality. When I was first diagnosed, I needed time to process everything. I wasn't ready to go public. I wanted it kept quiet. I didn't want people in the church to know about it just yet. But Mark, in his own method of processing, confidentially shared the news of my illness with his boss. His boss in turn shared it confidentially with his wife. She then shared it confidentially with someone else and off it went. Within hours it was public knowledge. It became spiritualized gossip. 'You should know this so you can pray,' was the theme. As a result, there were people who didn't talk to me at all because they knew they weren't supposed to know about my illness, and they didn't know how to act. It felt so awkward and uncomfortable. I felt violated. My right to privacy had been overlooked as people used prayer as a license to probe into delicate areas of my personal life. Their concern for me, which I do appreciate, however then led to undue curiosity, which then developed into a right-to-know attitude. The details of my illness became casual conversation. Because it didn't affect them personally, they weren't aware of the acuteness of its influence on me and the pain that it caused. While the intent was not to hurt me, they failed to consider my feelings. The lesson I learned from it was that I needed to be careful what I disclosed. Then I was criticized for not handling it well and being too private about my illness. That ticks me off!"

"Someone in the church said that I wouldn't make it to Tonya's high school graduation, too. I can't believe the careless statements that people make. They think those things won't get back to me, but they do."

Jennifer sat with her head down. Her body seemed to wilt as she described in detail different events. The light illuminating the room appeared to dim as though in response to her somber mood. Her eyes fixed on her hands that rested listlessly in her lap as the details fell from her lips in stoic rhythm. Straightening her back she emphatically stated, "It felt good to defy that prediction. It felt good to show them they were wrong. This struggle is hard enough without people overtly placing bets on how long I will last. Like the doctor in our congregation who said, 'She doesn't have a prayer.' Well, prayer is the one thing I do have going for me! Cut me some slack!"

Their comments were unknowingly cruel, driving each syllable into the marrow of Jennifer's spirit like an arrow piercing a straw target. They didn't recognize how devastating their idle talk was. It clung to her heart like crystal granules on a frosty window.

*Whatever leisure time we are able to invest in
relationships is time well spent."   - Charles R. Swindoll*

"The adventures have really been the best thing,"
Jennifer said as we pushed our empty plates to the other side
of the table. The view of the lake had disappeared and
nightfall had settled across the horizon. Except for the light
in the dining room, the rest of the lake house was dark.

"As a pastor and pastor's wife, we've had to be careful
not to get overly close to any one couple in our
congregation. We've learned that it isn't healthy and it just
doesn't work to have favorites within your church. But, at
the same time, we are people, too, and we need close friends
with whom we can be ourselves and be totally open and
honest. We've needed an outlet and we found that in you
guys. We've been friends for years, and because you aren't
part of our congregation, we can be more ourselves. It's
good to have best friends. We have loved our adventures,
primarily because we've been with you guys. It's
comforting to be with people with whom we can let our hair
down. We don't have any pretenses or images to keep up.
We can say and do pretty much whatever we feel like and
know that we are accepted."

"The other significant part of the adventures is that they
are fun. They take our minds off things. They give us
something to look forward to. There's maybe a whole week
or more where we prepare for an adventure and look
forward to it. Then there's the adventure itself. They've all
been different and they've been fun. Then there is the
afterglow as we reflect on the fun we had. It's such a nice
diversion from the pain and the routine that is so much a part
of our lives. They've all been good adventures, but the
wagon ride through Amish country was my favorite."

It had become increasingly difficult to come up with adventures in which Jennifer could participate. Our times together became less active. We usually arranged our adventures together, but the wagon ride had been a surprise for her. The plan was for Mark and Jennifer to come to our home for Sunday dinner and spend a quiet afternoon with us. After eating on the deck Rich said, "We planned something for us to do this afternoon."

"Great. What is it?" Mark responded.

"Well, you'll find out when we get there," Rich laughed.

"Okay! Let's do it," Jennifer returned as she jumped to her feet, unconcerned with what might be coming next.

We drove down the road a couple miles to Walt's house. Walt was warm, personable, and loved people. Although not tall in stature, he was large in spirit. He was a hard worker and always treated me well. Walt was a storyteller whose tales of when my parents and he were young gripped my attention. Walt had a wagon and a team of large fawn-colored workhorses. The horses were well mannered and as hospitable as Walt. Except for one being minutely bigger, they were identical, mirroring the white patch between their eyes that fell to their noses. Their manes and tails were blonde, an impressive contrast to their light tan backs. Walt was harnessing the horses when we arrived. We introduced our friends to each other, then watched Walt maneuver the horses into place in front of the wagon. Jennifer loved horses and she immediately fell in love with them and Walt.

"This is so neat," she told Walt. "This is just my speed. Usually they have me mountain climbing or something," she laughed. She jumped up onto the wagon and accepted her seat in front as the guest of honor alongside Walt. Slapping the reins and beginning his stories, Walt slowly drove the horses from his little farm nestled in the valley. We listened from behind, straining to catch each word. He told Jennifer about his horses and the history of the farms along the way. Jennifer snapped a picture of the horses from her seat as they pulled us along the roadway. The picture was later framed and held a special spot on the end table in her living room.

52

It was symbolic of, as she put it, "the best adventure we've ever had."

We turned onto a dirt road that wound its way through trees and hills, past creeks and homes with Amish buggies in side yards. We waved to bearded Amish men sitting in rocking chairs on their porches. Dark-clad children, who played like barnyard kittens, peered from behind fences and around the corners of houses. They interrupted their play to wave and watch as we clomped down the road. I could hear Jennifer quiz Walt about the Amish lifestyle. He answered her questions, weaving a storyline into each response.

From the distance I could see a small group of Amish children coming up the road on foot. Their dark clothes looked hot for such a warm afternoon. Bonnets were drawn loosely over brown wisps of hair. Their bare feet made prints in the soft dirt. As they reached us they smiled and waved. Walt stopped the wagon and talked with the youngsters he obviously knew. The youngest children aren't taught English right away, but they nonetheless communicated through their smiles and bright eyes. The group huddled around the wagon. A couple of the younger girls, intrigued by our lifestyle as much as we were by theirs, glanced at my sneakers, then my plaid shirt. Their eyes slowly followed to my hands, taking careful notice of my rings and polished fingernails. Timid faces smiled at me after checking out my earrings. Our lifestyles and language were worlds apart, yet we communicated through warm expressions and positive body language. We overcame the barriers of custom and tongue and came together to enhance each other's afternoon.

This was the same challenge for Jennifer and us; to somehow transcend the barriers her disease had created. Although at times we felt it had pushed us apart, we worked to overcome whatever obstacles tried to separate us. Too often clouds waited to overshadow our days and events. Sometimes we were successful in blasting them away but sometimes they surrounded us in a dark haze. We asked ourselves questions. When will it happen? How will it happen? Where will it be? How difficult will it be? How will I handle it? Jennifer and we all silently asked these same questions.

If you talk with the doctors, some may give you their estimate of the likely conditions that may surround the inevitable. They hesitate to give timeframes, but some make that guess. As far as I know, Jennifer asked only about the probable symptoms leading up to her demise – minimal pain, coma, death. She probably replayed that image in her mind. I know I did. It haunted me in a way that knit that visualization into every plan for every day I spent with her.

During one difficult evening huddled in the rocking chair in front of our fireplace, Jennifer asked the hard questions, but for her they ran root deep. Her heart was in no way rebellious or contrary, but one that was filled with pain. There was grief in her soft voice. Our compassion at that moment was merely a figure of speech as we were helpless to relieve her burden. The cares that pressed against her spirit could not be lifted. Her pain seemed beyond the power of our love to eliminate. I remained silent as Mark struggled to bring comfort through theological reason.

A slight wheeze made nearly every breath she took audible. She leaned forward in the chair to study the flames on the logs, then resolutely laid her head back and rocked rhythmically as she sat mesmerized by the fire. We wanted to shatter the impenetrable wall that separated the three of us from her. But it was solid and defiantly mocked all attempts to release her from the prison of her diagnosis.

"The Terminator," she said woefully in reference to God. "I want to see Him as my Healer, my Best Friend and my Comforter, but tonight He feels like The Terminator."

The image of her impending death hung stubbornly to the wall. At times the three of us assaulted the wall, wanting to snatch her away so things could return to normal. We wanted to pray hard enough and sustain a faith great enough that we could say to this mountain, "Be gone." But it was stubborn. It wouldn't go. We thought for a while that maybe the disease had gone, but it returned with such vengeance that my faith in healing was becoming as weak as she was physically. Sometimes my guilt was strong. Had I not prayed hard and long enough? Was I, in fact, sabotaging the effects of my prayers by my own shortcomings? What was the "right" combination of words and proper number of times to ask God for physical healing? How could we find the miraculous solution to release her from the verdict of death?

Jennifer tried to break through the wall also, yet her diagnosis held her captive. The shroud to the barrier was thick, firmly held in its place by the blood tests and MRI. We resigned to the fact that there was no formula to God's healing, only God's grace. We learned to recognize His goodness that surfaced through the difficult days. Sometimes for short periods we met at the wall that seemed to separate us and emerged together, all of us different and all carrying the stench of the shroud. Yet, we did emerge and in that emerging we discovered a deeper substance of life which, although painful, transcended the horror of terminal illness. There was a plane we ascended that overshadowed the grief – a place where we were always aware of the inevitable, yet deliberately laid it aside. We claimed the moment and captured every morsel of beauty and good we could. During those times soul pressed against soul and the future became only a myth. For in those moments there was no death, only life, life in its fullest and best. We laughed. We made plans for the future. We dreamed of the wonderful accomplishments we would achieve. We saw greater magnificence in sunsets and reflections of splendor in what we once had considered mundane. We dreamed our dreams and life stood still.

We continually planned for the future, not in a form of denial or refusal to accept the truth, but in a process to help Jennifer sustain her stamina. She needed adventures to plan for and talk about. They gave her something to think about beyond her symptoms.

We dreamed together on a bench in the middle of Eaton Centre in Toronto, at a beach on Lake Michigan, in a hotel lobby in Indianapolis. We dreamed of the store Jennifer would open for breast cancer patients. It would be unique, unlike the drab, impersonal places she'd been forced to shop for special helps since her mastectomy. Rather than a bleak reminder of breast cancer, she wanted her customers to experience the delight of their femininity at a time when they may not be feeling very feminine.

Hers would be a gracious and inviting store, a place of quiet pleasure. The décor would be refined. The walls would display artwork that expressed life and vitality. The details would be soothing and elegant, right down to the etched glass windows that would provide both light and privacy. The personal dressing rooms would be lavish with a comfortable settee that beckoned you to relax. Her store would bring hope and it would feel good to those entering within. It would be a respite from the realties of treatment. It was important to Jennifer that the new mastectomy patient investigate her current options in apparel with dignity.

The allure for her store increased as she described it. We could see it together as I felt the intensity of her vision. We became completely absorbed in her project and brainstormed names for the business. It'd been fun, but more importantly, it had been meaningful. It'd given her a vivid dream to hang onto. It was an admirable and worthwhile project that would not only bring her fulfillment, but also meet the needs of women facing the same struggles as she. It was an exciting dream. The fatigue melted from her face as we talked about it. Her eyes brightened and her shoulders straightened. An incredible energy seemed to flood her spirit as together we envisioned French doors, oriental rugs and pleased customers.

"Tonya can help me do it," she planned, "and it would be something for her later." A glowing pink hue returned to her cheeks. Her eyes sparkled and danced. Her voice was reflective as her mind reeled with ideas. It gave her a sense of purpose.

56

We cradled and nurtured her dream for months. She thought about it every day. It sustained and energized her. It gave her a link to the future.

CHAPTER 8   PRAYER FOR STRENGTH

"Friendship cheers like a sunbeam; charms like a good story; guides like a heavenly vision."   - Newell Dwight Hillis

"Look at the sky," Jennifer said, almost startled, as she looked out the window of the lake house. "Have you ever seen anything so beautiful? Look how the moon seems to be hanging over the lake, shining across the top of the waves. And look at all those stars. Isn't it a gorgeous night?"

"Humm," I responded as I stretched back in my chair, my back stiff from sitting so long. "It really is. Listen to the waves washing up on shore. It is so beautiful here. I love seeing the night sky and listening to the water."

Another beauty of that moment was that time just didn't matter. Our untethered interlude at the lake had disengaged us from the rest of the world.

"I can't believe how late it is," Jennifer laughed as she glanced at the clock.

"It's been a great day," I returned.

"It's been the best," she smiled.

Together we carried our dirty dishes to the kitchen and slowly yawned our good nights and headed for bed. Through my bedroom window I saw reflections of the late-night sky mirrored against the water. As I stood in the darkness I felt drawn to the rhythms of the water. I felt blessed to be there with Jennifer. She challenged me to live life more fully. Settling into my pillow I continued to reflect on good times that we'd shared. I thought about the dinners and cookouts. I remembered days at the beach flying kites and evenings watching orange sunsets. I thought about the Imax Theater. I laughed to myself recalling the evening the four of us relentlessly "interviewed" one of Tonya's new boyfriends while she dressed to go out on a date with him.

A kaleidoscope of sketches unfolded outlining our journal of experiences. I cherished each memory as sleep gradually overtook my body.

Sunlight soon flooded my room announcing a new day. I squinted to see what time it was and slowly rose from my bed. The sun was casting a white sheen over the water. I put on shorts and grabbed my sneakers, then quietly headed out the door for my morning walk. I moved briskly as I enjoyed the cool morning air. When I returned to the lake house I found Jennifer making coffee.

"Good morning," she chimed. "How was your walk?"

"Wonderful," I replied. "There's nothing nicer than a walk by the water in the morning. It's a beautiful day."

"It sure is. What should we have for breakfast?" she asked.

"Something simple. How about coffee, juice and cereal?" I responded.

"That sounds good to me," Jennifer said. "Let's eat on the table out by the lake."

I carried our tray of food as Jennifer held the door open for me. We ate leisurely and enjoyed the morning sunshine.

"How do you like your new home," I asked Jennifer.

"It's good," she replied. "I appreciate having everything on one floor. It was getting rather tough climbing all the stairs in our other house. Having the washer and dryer in the basement and our bedrooms on the second floor made laundry day hard. I did a lot of sitting on stairs in between floors to catch my breath. One day as I was sitting on the stairs half way to our bedroom with a pile of clean laundry in my lap I leaned back against the wall. I thought I'd just close my eyes for a minute to regain my strength. The next thing I knew the phone was ringing and I was wondering where in the world I was at. Apparently I had fallen asleep and when the phone rang I was so startled that I sent my lapful of clothes all over the stairway. Now that was rather annoying!" Jennifer laughed.

"Well, I guess," I responded. "So much for clean laundry. Mark told us that he had to carry you up to bed at night because climbing the stairs would sometimes leave you coughing and exhausted."

"He did do that," Jennifer continued. "The stairs became too difficult. I knew a move would be a good thing, but the packing nearly did me in."

"I knew that immediately when we arrived to help you." I replied. You sounded fine on the phone the day before the move but when we got there you didn't look so good. You really scared me."

"I did overdo it. I felt bad that I wasn't able to help with the actual move," she responded. "It was hard being that sick, leaving all the work for you guys."

"I had no doubt in my mind that it was difficult for you because you're not one to sit back and let others carry your load." I affirmed. "I knew you had to *really* be sick to let me and Tonya set up your kitchen without even supervising us."

I did a flashback to that New Years Day move. As Tonya and I unpacked the boxes of dishes and food items, she turned to me and said, "I don't think Mom could handle anyone else but you doing this. I'm glad you're the one helping us."

"Me, too," I responded to Tonya. I had wanted to cry and I was sure Tonya did too. In my heart I questioned if this was the beginning of the end. Would Jennifer pull out of this? Was the move, intended to make her life easier, going to be the element that pushed her beyond her physical limit and ushered in her death? I let Tonya make most of the decisions of where to put things in the kitchen that day. In my heart I feared Jennifer would never use that kitchen and it would, by default and necessity, become Tonya's kitchen. I figured she should be the one to make the final decisions.

Not long after the move Jennifer was alone in the house. She was still weak and unable to do much. A car drove up their street and pulled into their driveway. Jennifer recognized the woman who emerged from the vehicle. It was a lady who attended their church. She was not a close friend. In fact, she had never visited their home before. She seemed a bit apprehensive as she approached the door, but Jennifer dispelled any uneasiness by her greeting. They had talked for a few minutes when the woman told Jennifer that the Lord wanted her to pray for Jennifer. "He told me to pray for your strength," she explained.

Grateful for the prayers of those who sincerely believed God could change circumstances, Jennifer readily consented. The prayer was not lengthy nor philosophical in nature, but sincere and direct. After continued conversation, the woman excused herself and was gone. But, the effects of her prayer did not leave with her. Gradually and miraculously Jennifer began to feel better. Day by day as January progressed, Jennifer became stronger.

One day after being housebound for an extended period Jennifer impulsively called Mark at work and asked him to come home at noon so he could take her to get her hair cut. She became energized and excited as she began to do more and more. One of the first things she did was rearrange the kitchen I feared she would never use.

"I never thought it would feel so good to be able to wash dishes," she told me. "Washing them made me feel wonderful!" Each day she became stronger than she had been in two years.

I called to talk to her one evening and Mark explained that she was at the store buying some things in preparation for a trip she and Mike, their son, were taking. As impulsively as she had gotten her hair cut, she planned a trip. She was going home to see her mom and dad and all her friends and family. They left the following day. Her trip was a whirlwind of activity, visiting everyone she missed and loved. She spent an entire day at Disneyland also, walking from morning to night. As we got play-by-play reports of her activities, we were shocked and amazed beyond belief. Something miraculous certainly must have happened. We couldn't wait to see her after she returned home.

Her first day back we planned to have dinner together. When Rich opened our front door, Jennifer bounded energetically up the stairs from the foyer. "Look at you," I said astounded. I kept staring at her in amazement. "You look wonderful!"

The contrast was unbelievable. Her skin was clear and pink, all evidence of the jaundice gone. I couldn't see even a trace of yellow in the whites of her eyes. To see such resurgence of life within her was electrifying. She was effervescent as she enthusiastically replayed her whole trip, emphasizing the renewal of strength she'd experienced. "I don't know what's happening, but it sure has been good," she explained. "If I drop dead tomorrow, at least I've had a good month!"

Later in the restaurant I was aware that she hardly coughed, even though she was talking continually during our meal. As we returned to our car she tossed her head and began to skip with the freedom of a child. "Zip-a-dee-doo-dah, zip-a-dee-ay. My, oh, my what a wonderful day!" she sang. She was blessed and she knew it. She thanked God for His mercy and grace and each unencumbered breath.

Jennifer continued to do well. Although all traces of the disease had not disappeared, her energy level was high. She took part in activities she had put aside months earlier. We stepped back in wonderment to watch her animated personality. She was dynamic. Each day she looked for new evidence of a total recovery. She'd wake up in the morning and feel to see if the tumors on her head were shrinking. It seemed they might be. The possibility of experiencing a miraculous healing was exciting.

Our April adventure was the most expensive and elaborate one we'd ever planned. For weeks we considered and crafted our long weekend to see *The Phantom of the Opera* in Toronto. We purchased the music and familiarized ourselves with the storyline. We made reservations in a prominent downtown hotel, purchased box seat tickets and planned to have the most memorable adventure ever.

The week before we were to leave for Toronto, Rich and I sat in Mark and Jennifer's living room finalizing the details. We were so excited. This would be our best adventure yet. Telephone conversations throughout the week didn't reveal what I was soon to discover.

Their arrival at our home that early Friday morning to begin our trip together was heartbreaking. As Jennifer climbed out of their vehicle to greet us, she moved slower than usual. From the distance I saw that she seemed tired. Her face looked drawn and her expression subdued. When she approached to hug me, I saw it. The subtle hue from jaundice had returned to her complexion. The yellow in her eyes had returned and reflected a look of defeat. She hadn't wanted to tell me the remission had ended within the few days since I'd seen her. I clung to her not knowing what to say. There were no words to ease the moment. The disease was back to haunt us as treacherously as the phantom played out on the stage that weekend.

Jennifer and I rode in the backseat of the car, while the guys talked up front. I sat there dazed, trying to make small talk. She had used the days since I'd seen her to deal with it. She had needed that time to process what was happening. I now had to deal with it, not privately, but with her sitting two feet away from me. I was instantly angry with Mark for not telling me what was going on with her. I don't like surprises and it felt at that moment like he could and should have told me. "Why couldn't he have picked up the stupid phone and let me know?" I thought to myself. "This is no way to start an exceptional adventure." I looked out my window fighting the sadness from my face and rehearsed what I would say to Mark apart from Jennifer. I was angry and disappointed, although my emotions were really because the disease had manifest itself again. Mark became the object of that anger, though, because I had no place else to direct it. I seethed inside as we traveled further toward Toronto. Miles down the road, though, I concluded that Mark also had his own measure of processing to do. Letting him have it wouldn't change anything except to get him ticked off at me and put a damper on our weekend.

It took me a while, but I finally promised myself that we would reclaim this adventure. I wouldn't vent my disappointment on Mark and we wouldn't let the phantom break us against rocks of discouragement. We would not let him dominate our adventure. We would not be tormented by his horrible face.

After arriving in Toronto we checked into our hotel, which was only a short walk away from the theater. It was a wonderful facility with over 1,500 guestrooms, two restaurants and three lounges. We chose a restaurant near the hotel for dinner. We walked the streets slowly, investigating the variety of shops and restaurants along the way. We faked interest in store windows and moderated our speed so Jennifer wouldn't get tired out.

Saturday was theater day, the pinnacle of weeks of planning. As we sat in our private box seats awaiting the beginning of the performance, we agreed we were living out our perfect adventure in style. We were enraptured from the first eerie chords of Andrew Lloyd Webber's *Phantom* theme song to the final curtain bow of the cast.

The essence of the story revolved around difficult choices the cast of characters had to make in the midst of tragedy and beauty. As we left the opera house I was struck with the reality that we had to work through our own complex drama. We longed desperately for the adversary to be eradicated as effectively as it had been in the play. We prayed hard for a happy ending to our story.

"I have seen what a laugh can do. It can transform almost unbearable tears into something bearable, even hopeful.
- Mark Hope

The sun rose high in the clear morning sky. Only two small clouds hovered on the western horizon of the lake.

"It is getting hot," Jennifer said pushing her lawn chair back from our breakfast table. I'd really love to take one of those inner tubes and float around in the water."

I responded with the tone of my voice dropping on my last two words. "Yeah, that would really feel good, wouldn't it?" The potential danger of her idea had hit me mid-sentence.

"I'm not sure I'm strong enough to swim very far, though, if I were to fall out of the inner tube," Jennifer returned.

I was thankful she had recanted her thought. Although I could swim well, I would never have been able to live with myself if she fell into the water and I was unable to save her.

"Let's take our chairs to the water's edge and just splash our feet," I suggested.

"Good plan," she said and together we carried our chairs to the shoreline.

"Your shirt is so cute," I said to Jennifer. "That must be new. I've never seen it before."

"It is," she responded. "Most of my clothes have gotten too baggy since I've lost so much weight. I had to get some new things. I'm back to my pre-children size again. It feels good. I like how I look in this new version of myself. It reminds Mark of how I looked when we were first married."

"Well, you must have been a stunning bride," I said. "You'll have to show me your wedding album sometime."

"I sure will. I'd love to," Jennifer returned. Her voice softened then she slowly began. "You know, Anna, I told Mark the other night that I wanted him to get married again."

"Really?" I replied. I was a bit stunned by her comment. "Why did you tell him that?"

"Well," she continued, "we were talking about the journey I am on. We talked about how we have been together on this path in life for nearly 24 years. We went through the Army together, school, various churches. We had children. It's been great. Around every corner was some new unknown adventure waiting for us and we experienced everything together. But what's happening now is that we are traveling different roads. We came to a fork in the road and neither one can know what the other is experiencing. I'm on my own journey now, one that he can't understand. He has no idea what my journey is like. He can't relate to it."

"We believe mine will be the greatest adventure. We talked about what it will be like when I enter Heaven, when I see Jesus, when I see friends and family who have gone before me. We tried to picture in our minds what was around the bend for me."

"Then we talked about the road he was traveling. We talked about the fact that he would be alone. I don't want him to be alone. It won't be good for him. I told him that it would be okay if one day he might find and love someone else. That doesn't threaten me. It would be the right thing for him. He should get married again."

"Jen, I'm really impressed," I said. "I'm not sure I could do that. You actually have given him your blessing to find another woman. Plus, you also bought new furniture for him."

"Yes, I did. I bought the furniture because our other furniture wouldn't work for a bachelor. The colors were too light and just wouldn't be appropriate for him after I'm gone."

"Jen. I don't know what to say," I continued. "You deliberately think very specifically about him going forward. That's commendable. You are so mature and selfless. He is lucky to have you as his wife. He doesn't even begin to know what a gem he has!"

"I love him," she responded. "I want him to be happy. I want him to have a good life. I think his ministry will be more effective also with a good wife."

"He has a good wife, Jennifer. So, tell me, what's it like being a preacher's wife?" I asked as I leaned back in my chair.

"It's no different than being married to any other guy I guess," she returned. "Men are men and jobs are jobs. The difference comes, I think, from church people's expectations of the preacher's family. They sometimes put you on a pedestal and somehow expect you to be perfect."

"And you're not perfect?" I laughed.

"You, of all people, should know that I'm not. But to be successful, you try to maintain the image the church expects of you. Now, I'm not talking about moral expectations. That's a given. It's the little things that people can expect that sometimes can be difficult. You're expected to maintain the perfect home, have perfect kids, entertain guests at the drop of a hat, be an excellent cook, play the piano and a hundred other things. It's hard to be all things to all people."

Jennifer started laughing as she continued. "One time we were getting ready to move to another church. I had started to pack up the parsonage. I took everything out of my dresser drawers and had my bras and underwear lying out all over the bed. I had boxes of stuff sitting around and the place looked pretty messy. Well, right in the middle of all this the kids wanted to go to the beach. Part of me said that I shouldn't leave the mess but another part of me said to go for it. I figured that the kids probably wouldn't get to go to the ocean again because of the move, so I left everything and took them. When we got back and I started working at clearing the mess, I saw a car pull into the driveway. It was the parsonage committee from the church who needed to inspect the parsonage prior to our move. However, they hadn't told me they were coming and they just dropped in unannounced. They expected, of course, that would be fine because a pastor's house is always immaculate, right? Why would they need to give us any advanced notice for a house inspection?"

"I was panicked because the parsonage looked so horrible. I didn't know what to do. I didn't want anybody seeing the house looking that way, especially the parsonage committee. I didn't have a lot of time to think, so my first thought was that I just wouldn't answer the door. That'd work. They'd think I wasn't home and leave and that'd buy me some time to pull things together. So I grabbed the kids and quickly explained to them that we needed to be very quiet. We huddled out of sight while these people kept knocking and knocking and knocking. I didn't think there'd be any paint left on the door the way they were hammering on it. Finally they stopped knocking, but then I heard them wandering around the yard. I kept thinking, 'give it up, go away, come back later.' At last they concluded that I must not be home and started to leave. They got back in their car and began to drive out the driveway. I gave such a huge sigh of relief. I was so proud of myself for postponing the inspection. Just as I began to relax though I noticed Mark's car drive up just in time to meet their car. He waved out his window and they returned to our yard."

"Oh, Jen," I laughed. "What lousy timing! What happened? Did he let them in?"

"Well, sure he did," she continued laughing. "I could hear him talking to them in the yard saying, 'Come on in. I'll show you around.' I was absolutely, totally horrified. I didn't know what to do. I didn't want them to know that I really was home and hadn't answered the door. Again, I had to think fast. I told the kids to pretend like they had been sleeping, then I ran into the bedroom and hid in the closet. I could hear Mark come in and ask Mike where I was. Mike was such an actor. He stretched and yawned and said through his yawn something like 'Maybe she went to the store.' That was good. After all, **maybe** I did go to the store. And then again, **maybe** I didn't. Did I just put my son in the position of evading the truth? My mind was reeling too fast to get caught up in semantics. 'Oh, what a tangled web we weave . . . .' was my haunting thought!"

"I heard the voices of the members of the committee talking with Mark as he took them room by room through the parsonage. The voices suddenly got louder as everyone came into the bedroom. Mark was both shocked and embarrassed to see my underwear displayed all over the bed with everything else in such a mess. He regretted inviting them inside. Then the worst happened. I didn't think it could get worse, but it did. They started talking about the water pipe in the closet wall that had previously leaked. My heart started to beat wildly and I nearly fainted when I heard one of the committee members say that they should check to make sure that the pipe wasn't leaking again. I could hardly breathe. I didn't know what to do. I was certain they'd be able to hear my heart pounding in my chest. The sound seemed to echo off the walls inside that closet. I thought I was going to throw up. It was one thing to have to explain why the bedroom was such a wreck and another to explain why I hadn't answered the door. But, how in the world was I ever going to explain why I was in that closet?!"

Jennifer's laughter was explosive as she continued. "I heard footsteps come closer to the closet. I froze. I held my breath when the closet door suddenly came open. I saw Mark's face peer in. He squinted then flinched when he saw me standing there. He turned white. I don't know whose face had the greatest pathetic look of horror, his or mine. I could see the maze of silent questions disfigure his face as he wondered what the heck I was doing in that closet. He was pale, then suddenly his face flushed. He looked like he was going to pass out. He slammed that door shut so fast I thought it was going to come off the hinges. I could hear him stammering and stuttering. Finally I heard him say that everything was all right in the closet! Their voices quickly trailed out of the bedroom as he got rid of them as fast as he could. When he returned to the closet to give me the 'all clear sign' he just stood there smirking as I peeked out from behind the clothes. 'Nice, he said. Really nice.'"

Jennifer and I laughed until I thought we couldn't laugh any more, and then she got us going again. "See what I mean about being a pastor's wife. It's not easy!!!"

"You're something else," I giggled.

"You know, I really used to be fun before I got sick," she came back.

"I don't think being sick has hurt your sense of humor any," I laughed.

Time moved rapidly through our week at the lake. We laughed. We cried. We spent evenings watching the sun fall out of sight leaving a warm glow on the water. We took pictures trying to capture the illusion of holding the setting sun in our hands. We looked at the moon illuminating the nights' sky and spent hours creating memories that will live with me forever. We extended our time together when Jennifer asked if I could stay a little longer at the lake. Neither of us wanted this adventure to end.

Summer quickly advanced following our vacation. June soon became July bringing with it quiet excursions and Jennifer's fading strength. We shared casual dinners at home, grilled pork chops at the beach and flew our kites. Jennifer drank nutritional supplements in addition to her food in an effort to sustain her weight and energy, but she continued to become dangerously thin. Dropping pounds used to be a celebration, but no longer. She was aware there was no longer any reserve weight.

Her love for horses was evident as she accepted invitations from friends at the church to come to their farm to ride their horses. She lacked the strength to mount by herself, but they helped lift her into the saddle. She was tenacious and with everything within her she continued to experience life in its fullest.

Sitting at the beach one evening waiting for the pending sunset I asked her, "Do you still think about your store?"

"Every day," she smiled. "Every day."

We both knew that the store would never be a reality, but the vision was so strong and comforting to her that we continued to fantasize about it. As the sun began to settle on the horizon, Mark and Rich returned from their bike ride.

Mark grabbed the camera and took a picture of Jennifer and me sitting on the sand with the sun setting between us.

"What a beautiful sunset," Jennifer softly said. "They don't get any better than this."

We didn't know it then, but that was our final sunset and adventure together. On September 12, just twelve weeks following our time at the lake house, Jennifer experienced her ultimate adventure, and this time she went alone. The adventure brought brutal, searing pain, not for Jennifer, but for those she left behind - those who loved her most. The pain was deeper than all measure of expression.

I prayed through my tears, "Welcome her well, Lord. Please welcome her well." I envisioned her waking up from her coma and finding herself alive and whole, totally embraced by God. In my mind's eye I could see Him tenderly transforming her brokenness into joy. I visualized her instantaneous change from struggling for each breath to now inhaling deeply and fully with perfect new lungs. I found comfort in the fact that her suffering had ended and her soul was in heaven.

As I stood alongside Jennifer's casket prior to her funeral, I didn't take the picture she had glibly suggested, but I tearfully reflected on our friendship and adventures. Words cannot bring to life the value of our shared friendship. Although this chapter of our lives had come to a close, it will never come to an end. I can never let go of the impact Jennifer made on my life and the lessons she taught me. My friendship with her didn't define who I was, but it definitely enhanced who I was becoming.

Charles Dickens described it well when he said, "It was the best of times; it was the worst of times."

CHAPTER 10   ACCIDENTAL MEETING

"It isn't the big pleasures that count the most; it's making a great deal out of the little ones."   *- Jean Webster*

A year after Jennifer's death, Rich and I went camping at the lake. We spent the night with our tent pitched in the sand just a few feet from the edge of the water. I awoke to the sounds of sea gulls overhead and waves splashing against the shore. But my attention to those pleasant morning noises was soon diverted to the ache in my back.

"Who's idea was this," I mumbled to myself as I rolled over and realized that my air mattress had sprung a leak during the night. Every part of me hurt as I crawled to push back the tent flap to see the morning haze over the water. I slowly made coffee and moaned with each sip as Rich and I sat on the beach and discussed our plans for the day.

"Let's just keep it simple, okay?" I muttered. "My back won't take a twenty mile bike ride right now."

"That's fine with me," Rich returned. "My back isn't feeling so great either. I think this tent camping is for the birds. What do you say we exchange the tent and air mattresses for a motel room. We can leave the water running in the bathroom and pretend it's waves on the shore if you want to."

"I've got a good imagination," I smiled. "I think that will work. Let's do it!"

After breakfast, a quick shower and a stop at the ice cream stand, we began to walk along the beach. It was late morning. Hot summer days brought the people to these beaches, but a new season had begun. School had started. The lifeguards had returned to college and families were settled into new routines. The shoreline boasted a few sun worshippers indulging themselves in the fleeting rays of summer, but for the most part, the beaches were vacant. Occasionally, a biker would ride by on the pathway, only momentarily distracting our gaze at the water. In the distance a plump mom in a modest bikini played in the sand with her young children.

As I cocked my head to catch dripping ice cream on the side of my cone, I saw a man walking toward us. I turned to get a better look and saw Mark's familiar outline approaching. We hadn't seen him in many weeks. His hair was longer than I'd ever seen it and he looked tired. The lines in his forehead had deepened and I noticed that his temples had started to gray.

"Heh," came his cheerful greeting. "How are you guys doing?"

"We're doing good," Rich responded. "What a surprise. How are you? What's been happening with you and the kids?"

After catching up on the details of our lives, Mark turned to me. As tears filled his eyes he said, "Do you know what day this is?"

"Yes, I do," I responded, then looked down at my watch. I was surprised at the time and realized that it was one year ago that exact moment that Jennifer had left us. I was overcome with emotion.

"I knew you would remember," he said. "The kids and I bought flowers. I've been walking and reminiscing about her life."

There were miles of beaches along that lake. What were the odds of our running into Mark like that? It did make sense, though, that we be together right then to remember Jennifer.

"It's been a difficult year," Mark began.

"For all of us," I responded. "To be honest, the pain was so great that there were times I wished we had never met you guys. But the fragrance of our friendship was so strong in our hearts that I wondered what we'd be today had we not experienced it. I miss Jennifer. I miss her brave attempt to live life to the fullest and see the bright side of things on even the darkest days. I miss her gentle spirit seeking to please God and honor Him through her life and her death. I know you miss her too. What was the hardest part of this year for you?"

Mark's voice was irregular and he spoke almost in a whisper. His eyes were sad as he began. "The hardest part was that I was totally alone. As you know, the kids were about four hours away from me by that time. I remember going home and it felt so empty there. Before Jennifer went into the hospital she used to lie on the couch. I had my recliner beside the couch so we could watch TV together. I would look over at Jennifer to see how she was doing. She usually slept. She wasn't awake a lot at the last. I'd reach over and pat her. After she died I couldn't get that image out of my mind. I'd go home and sit in my chair and look over and she wasn't there. That was a very difficult period."

Mark's voice began to quiver as he continued. "I was very much alone. I had friends – people from the church that either called or stopped by. You and I spoke on occasion but at that time, you guys were several hours away also. I talked to the kids. People tried to comfort me. It wasn't that no one reached out. They did. But it was at night after 9:00 o'clock when the house was quiet and empty that there were haunting memories. I would remember helping Jennifer to bed and her lying there. I would remember her frail body in the bathtub taking a baking soda bath because she was in pain. I remembered the last time we had sex. Those memories were so vivid. They were SO VIVID," Mark emphasized. "They haunted me." His voice softened then grew strong and loud. "They haunted me. They HAUNTED me!!! It seems like you don't know at the time that this will be the last time you're going to do or say or feel things. Then when the death occurs, that's when they become the last things that happened and you tend to remember them. They just stick in your mind. What was the hardest part for you?"

"Going on," I responded. "We had to go on, and we did, each in our own way. Jennifer's struggle was over, but I

74

was overwhelmed by my own struggle. Prior to Jennifer's death a wall separated her and the rest of the world because no one could fully relate to what she was going through. Following her death it seemed that a wall was separating me from the rest of my world because no one could really relate to what I was feeling. It certainly was unlike the lonely walk Jennifer had traveled yet the depths of the solitude left my soul dormant. I don't think Rich even fully realized the extent of the seclusion I sometimes felt."

"In helping Jennifer dream her dreams, unconsciously and without realizing it, her dreams had become my dreams and when she died, my dreams died too. It suddenly felt very empty. My focus in life for so long had been helping her get through her difficult journey. Now the focus was over and some of those around me didn't understand why I shouldn't be over it too. After all, I knew it was coming, didn't I? Jennifer's death shouldn't have been a surprise to me, but it was. She had rallied so many times before, I thought maybe she would that time too. In countless ways she seemed invincible in my mind. I should have been prepared, but I wasn't. I should have expected the suffocating pain I felt, but I didn't. I functioned and I went on, but there was an empty grieving hole in me that wouldn't go away."

"I remember I took the week of Thanksgiving off to prepare for the holidays and begin my Christmas shopping. I figured that keeping busy would ease the pain. I drove to the shopping mall within a few miles from where you guys had lived. I wandered through stores looking for gifts but I felt distanced from everything and everybody. I gave it up and drove to Barnes and Noble, which you know is usually a fix for me when I'm down. I walked the aisles looking at hundreds of books stacked neatly on the shelves but they were uninviting as though void of content and meaning, just covers with bare pages. So I got in my car and headed for the beach where we all had shared our last adventure together. The wind off the lake put a chill in my bones. The waves were gray, churning up black weeds on the shoreline.

The beaches were empty and the sand was strewn with sticks and driftwood. The tall stark trees were a silhouette of loneliness. They were as empty and bare as I felt. The beach seemed to be a mirror of my soul. Another season had taken over the beach and another season had taken over my life and I could hardly stand it."

"When I decorated the house for Christmas I pulled out the red Christmas tins that Jennifer had given the kids the previous Christmas. You remember how she had made chocolate chip cookies and placed them inside for the boys. As sick as she was, she wanted to give them something from her for Christmas. You know, small cookie crumbs still remain in the bottom of those tins. I couldn't bring myself to wash them out because there on the bottom of the tins, now stale with age, are the remnants of Jennifer's expression of love. They represent her precious energy spent and they are cherished."

"Was it a surprise for you when she died, Mark?" I asked.

The three of us settled on a picnic table on the beach as we continued talking. Mark looked out across the water as he responded.

"Yes, I was surprised. I remember getting the phone call that night saying Jennifer had gone into a coma. I didn't expect that. She was in the hospital – one of the safest places she could have been. She was better off there than she was at home. /She went in for a routine, very simple, minor procedure. There was no indication that her organs were going to fail and that she would slip into a coma. We had no inkling whatsoever. We just thought she would go into the hospital, get some relief and come home and linger on for months and months and months. So, when I got the call and they said something like 'It looks like this may be it. We've called the doctor. (Mark's voice breaks.) We think you ought to call your family,' I was shocked. Tonya and I jumped up, got dressed, and ran to the car. All the way to the hospital we were in tears and in shock. So, yeah, it was a surprise. I didn't expect that."

"I wished I had stayed with Jennifer that last night she was in the hospital. I didn't realize that she was so far gone. I didn't realize she would go into a coma that night. I remember so vividly. Tonya and I were visiting her and visiting hours were up. They were going to change her sheets because she had gotten a lot of blood on them. They asked us to leave while they changed the sheets. Jennifer said, 'Well, why don't you guys go on home.' I remember walking out of the room and going down to the elevator and looking back and seeing Jennifer looking out the door."

Great emotion filled Mark and his voice shook erratically as he continued. ". . . . . . . and something in me said I ought to stay, but I didn't." Tears stream down his face as he looks intently at Rich. "Rich, ... I didn't stay. I should have stayed but I left and went home. I regret not being there during her last conscious hours. I regret that very much."

Mark's sobbing continued and then he straightened his arms across the top of the picnic table. His voice took a hard, firm tone. "I also regret, and will to my dying day . . . . . that I wasn't beside her when she died. I have such guilt about that. I stepped out to make a phone call and a nurse came and told me that she was gone. I will never forgive myself for that. Not that she would have known I was there, but . . . . . I regret that."

A slight breeze began to blow and rippled the water on the lake as Mark collected his emotions. The sun was warm against our faces. "What are some things that you are glad you did?" Rich asked.

"Oh . . . . I'm glad that we went to see Kenny Rogers," Mark returned with a slow smile on his face. It was a great moment for Jennifer and me – a great memory. She was pretty sick and weak at the time. It was winter. Mike bought the tickets to the concert as a gift to his mother. She really wanted to see Kenny Rogers. We got there early. Of course, you know how she was about being in a wheelchair. She was embarrassed. It was a little embarrassing to wheel her into the auditorium."

"Why was it embarrassing for you to wheel her in the wheelchair?" I asked.

"Well, it was embarrassing for both of us," he replied. "Jennifer was embarrassed because she didn't like to be stared at in the way people sometimes do with people in a wheelchair. I think we all want to be looked at and admired, respected and even envied in a sense. That's why we try to look our best. There's a sense of adrenaline that pumps through you when you get all dressed up and go out. You want to be seen at your best. Yet, when you're not at your best, when you are perceived as somehow weak or sick, you don't want people to see you. You don't want to be pitied. You don't want to be looked down upon, and you definitely don't want to be rejected. Those were all the things we were feeling at that time. People look at you differently when you are in a wheelchair. Nobody wants to be in that position where you're looked at differently – especially rejected. People don't mean to reject you, but they reject you in so many different ways. They look at you and then they look away. They don't speak to you in the same way that they would speak to you normally if you were standing at eye level."

"I can remember that night at Kenny Rogers; we did get there early, earlier than most people. There was a crowd lined up already waiting to get in and get their seats. Because Jennifer was in a wheelchair, we had made arrangements for her to go out on the floor first, so I had to roll her through the vestibule to get to the elevator. People just stared. I mean it was a natural reaction on their part but it was also a natural reaction on our part that we didn't want to be looked at. It was embarrassing. It wasn't until we got to our seats and we put the wheelchair away that we felt totally normal again, because now we were just like everybody else. We were sitting in our seats waiting for the concert."

"Then Kenny Rogers came out and it was a real intimate, special time for us because Jennifer loved Kenny Rogers. He was one of her favorite singers. It was the first time we had ever gone to a concert together. It was a wonderful moment. I remember I sat with my arm around her. She was weak and frail. I felt protective. She was very yellow, as you recall, but she felt pretty good that night. She just beamed. It was one of her better nights. She didn't wheeze and cough a lot, even though she was weak. It was a good night. I was glad I did that right," Mark laughed. "It was a good night."

Mark's mood had lightened and his shoulders were more relaxed. The stress lines left his face and he seemed at ease talking with us. We were thankful we had run into him.

"What was the most meaningful adventure for you that the four of us shared?" Rich asked.

"Oh, I think Toronto was spectacular," he replied with a large smile. "No doubt, that was the best time, don't you think?"

"It was great, after I got over being mad at you," I teased.

"I know, I know," he smiled. "It really was terrific though. I had thought about going to see the Phantom for about a year. Then we actually did it. We went to a glamorous hotel, ate out, went to the play, and had box seats. It was probably the most elegant time I'd ever experienced. Jennifer and I never did a lot of fancy stuff. When we were in Santa Cruz we were surrounded by a lot of rich people and occasionally they would ask us out to these exclusive places. But, we always felt uncomfortable. That's not who we were. We were just regular people. But going to Toronto with you guys, we felt kind of cool."

"It was very neat," Rich replied.

"That was a real adventure," Mark emphasized. "It was exciting and I loved it. I'll always remember back to that time. The bond of friendship the four of us shared was strong. Since Jennifer's death and my move, it is one of the things I have really missed."

"We've missed it, too, Mark. We've missed it too," Rich affirmed.

"A friend is one who joyfully sings with you when you're on the mountain top, and silently walks beside you through the valley."   - William A. Ward

"Mark, what were your initial thoughts and feelings when Jennifer was diagnosed as terminally ill," Rich asked.

Mark paused to reflect thoughtfully, then began. "I remember being there with Jennifer at the doctor's office and nervously waiting for the doctor to come in. He was very kind, patient, gentle. He basically just diagnosed. He told Jennifer that the cancer had metastasized and he told her where it was located. When asked if there was anything that we could do, he said, 'No, it is terminal.' When I heard that word terminal I was shocked. I mean, I heard the diagnosis. I heard all the parts of the body, but then when I heard the word terminal, there was a disconnect. Somehow I thought with modern medicine and everything available today there must be something we could do."

"I remember being blown away, but Jennifer seemingly was in perfect peace. It was such an amazing thing. I think she already knew. She was very much in tune with her own body and knew something was radically wrong. She had already guessed the seriousness of this illness and knew what the outcome would be. She told the doctor she had peace about it. She said she didn't want to go to extraordinary lengths with medical procedures. There were a few things she could have pursued. He offered some preliminary suggestions, but she declined them and said she was going to trust God with the outcome."

"Following the doctor visit, Jennifer was fairly upbeat in terms of her faith that God might possibly heal her. She never said for certain that He would. She never made any claims like that. She did believe in supernatural healing and

I think at that moment she was fairly positive about the possibility for that happening."

"What about later?" I asked. "Do you feel she maintained that peace?"

"I don't know all that Jennifer shared with you," Mark began, "but remarkably in the nineteen months from the diagnosis to the time she died, I can only remember about two times she was ever down or the least bit depressed. Both times were primarily when Jennifer came to the realization that she wasn't going to get well and that God wasn't going to heal her. She wept primarily for the things she was going to miss, like the kids' weddings, grandchildren and stuff like that. But, incredibly, those are the only times I ever saw her down. Even in the moments she was the sickest, in the most pain and was totally wracked with those coughing jags she used to have, as you recall, she never felt sorry for herself. She never got depressed. She never lost her love or intimacy with God. As a matter of fact, she drew closer to Him."

"Actually, as a family, we were all pretty upbeat. We thought that Jennifer would somehow get through this. I mean, we knew that it was terminal. That's where I know some people would think this was a total disconnect. You hear the doctor say it's terminal so you have that kind of scientific evidence on the one hand, but on the other hand we were people of faith. We did believe in miracles and who better than a person like Jennifer for God to heal. There was a measure of optimism within our family. Now I will say this: as time went on, Jennifer was more positive and upbeat on her end than I was. I ultimately accepted the fact that the prognosis would come to pass. I mean, I was dealing with that more so than she was. I thought it was a long shot that God would heal her, let's put it that way."

"I know this is not something you can definitively answer," I responded, "but how much of that was faith and how much do you suppose it might have been denial – protecting herself from reality?"

Mark shifted in his seat and smoothed the surface of the sand with his foot before he responded. "I'm sure from a psychological standpoint, if a psychiatrist or a psychologist was to have examined Jennifer, they would have called it denial. But, Anna, I believe that it was faith. I believe what I saw in Jennifer was genuine faith because it was so positive. It was so joy filled. She was so much at peace. A psychologist will tell you that you go through stages of grief, and denial is one of the first stages. Then you move on to those other stages. Jennifer didn't pass through all those stages. She didn't get angry. She wasn't like that at all that I saw. Now maybe she told you things other than what I experienced. In living with her day to day I saw genuine faith. And what I saw even more than that was an accelerated growth in her relationship with God. I can remember I actually envied the intimacy that I saw in Jennifer's walk with the Lord the last year of her life. She was depending on Him in a way that most of us don't understand and don't know how. I mean, she was depending on God for every breath she was taking, in a very real sense. It was marvelous. It was wonderful to see. So, it's a perspective thing. If you have eyes of faith, you will see faith in action. If you don't have eyes of faith, you're going to say it's denial. That's how I would explain it."

"I buy that," I responded. "She had a very mature faith. On another note, tell me your perspective about the things people said that hurt her."

Mark leaned forward and watched a sea gull run along the shore. "Well," he began, "there are two that stand out in my mind. First there were people of faith who had all kinds of advice and all kinds of books they had read that had been meaningful to them. They thought Jennifer ought to either try the advice or read the book. Basically it was, 'If you do this, then God will do this.' We were not into that 'name it – claim it' kind of stuff. You know that. The four of us talked about some of that over the course of time. So, often times when these people would come with those kinds of solutions, it was offensive to us. We didn't appreciate it.

We knew they meant well, but we didn't believe like that. That's not how we organized our life or our faith. So we had on the one hand what I call the religious zealots that went to our church. They were sometimes disturbing although they were all nice, well-meaning people."

"Then, on the other hand, there were well-meaning people with medical solutions. One of the reasons we went back home following Jennifer's diagnosis was not only to share with her mom and dad the fact that she had terminal cancer, but also somebody had lent us a beach house. We went there and spent a couple days just to map out what we were going to do."

"The man who owned the beach house was a doctor. We had mutual friends who had been in a former church. The doctor and his mutual friend came to the beach house. The friend had a rare cancer that she felt she had beaten but it had required a heroic effort. The woman described the horrific pain she went through. It was a complicated procedure and very experimental. The insurance companies weren't paying for it. It was a last-gasp measure. They couldn't understand why Jennifer wouldn't apply for it. Interestingly enough, the lady who was advocating this procedure died shortly after Jennifer died. She had spent thousands upon thousands of dollars for her medical treatment. The last year of her life was spent in hospitals whereas Jennifer's was spent at home enjoying her friends and family."

"Jennifer and I talked and one thing we didn't want was for her illness to wreck the finances of the family and totally ruin us. We talked about that a lot because we had known families who could not accept the inevitable. They went to desperate measures that in the process destroyed themselves, their family, and their finances. We determined not to do that."

"So, to answer your question, we had people that had a religious solution and then we had the medical people. Again, all were very well-meaning people. Then, if the truth were known, we had another situation where the people weren't so well meaning. Jennifer was being treated by a cancer clinic and had told the doctor the first day she went in, 'I'm not really interested in pursuing the chemo and radiation. I've gone that route. I've had chemotherapy and it made me deathly sick and I don't want to spend the rest of what short time I have left going through all those medical procedures. All I am interested in is getting palliative care.'"

I could hear the anger building in Mark's voice as he continued. "Well, the doctor rejected that and as a result, he rejected Jennifer. When it came right down to the point where she needed some kind of shot to take away the pain and the itching, he refused to give it to her because she would not follow his prescribed methods. Radiation, chemo, and all that harsh stuff would have done her no good whatsoever!"

The volume in Mark's voice was increasing and his words accelerated as he literally seemed to spit them out. "I remember very distinctly that she was hurting badly. I took her in to the cancer clinic but they wouldn't even see her. They would do nothing for her. I was so angry with the doctors at that clinic. I've never been angrier in my life. That was such a lousy thing to do to her!"

Mark's voice calmed as he paused to collect himself and then continued. "Those were some of the irritating things. Also Jennifer's sister saw Jennifer's acceptance of her illness as somehow giving up. Jennifer was at peace with it. She had faith in God. She was trusting in God to take care of her. If God wanted her healed, she believed God would heal her. But she wasn't going to go to extraordinary lengths and go through all those medical procedures only in the end to come to the same place. But her sister was not a person of faith and she saw Jennifer's attitude as giving up. I can remember Jennifer having discussions with her about it. I think she came away a little bit hurt because she felt that she had come to terms with her illness and she was at peace with it. She was doing what a woman of faith would do, but her sister saw it as quitting. 'Look we can fly you any place in the world to get treatment' she'd say. People gave all kinds of advice and cures and interpreted her walk of faith as failure to fight the cancer. That was very painful to her. I think it wasn't the case at all. I saw it as courage. She possessed a great deal of an inner strength."

Mark's words expressed intense emotion. They were fast and deliberate. "It wasn't desperate. I saw my father. I know what my father went through when he died. He was not a man of faith and he went to desperate measures to stay alive and there was no peace there at all. It was not a pretty sight. It was just the opposite of what Jennifer went through and how she handled it. I say often that I learned so much from Jennifer watching her go through that. I'll take those lessons with me to the grave. I hope and I pray that I can respond to my demise as she did. It was such a heroic acceptance of what she experienced."

"A very difficult time for me was when we traveled to tell her parents and my mom that Jennifer had terminal cancer. When Jennifer told my mom, my mom broke down weeping and went over to Jennifer and embraced her. That's what you would expect. That's what you would want. This was a tragedy. But when she told her parents, it was like – okay, and how are the kids? It was almost that nonchalant. It was such a contrast. That's how they took the news of their daughter's terminal illness. I couldn't believe it. Now you have to know them. They are very private people. There is no hint of weakness in them. I remember detesting her mom and her dad because they were so stiff upper lipped and hardly responded to the information. I was so angry with them over their apathy that I couldn't even sleep in their house that night. I went over to my mom's and spent the night there."

"It was stupid of me. I should have been there to support Jennifer. She knew I was angry with them, but she loved her parents and was very defensive of them. It was a source of conflict for Jennifer and me during that time, to be honest. I was mad at her parents right up to the day that Jennifer died. I had certain expectations that were not met. I expect people to respond in a certain way probably because it's the way I respond to things. I tend to be a tenderhearted person, and my initial reaction is one of putting my arms around a hurting person to comfort and console them. It's just so natural to me. That was my expectation of them. I thought when we went there they would do that and when they didn't, it was a very difficult thing to witness and accept."

"Now later, they had talks and her parents expressed their love for Jennifer. They expressed their pain for her loss and their loss. They made a trip to the lake house in August just prior to Jennifer's death. The family was all together. They celebrated Jennifer's last birthday with her there. But I didn't go. I was still very angry with her whole family. Jennifer wanted me to go. I didn't want to go. That's probably another regret I have. I didn't know that was the last time the family was going to get together. However, I know that when Jennifer came back from that time with her family she had gotten everything she wanted from them – the tenderness, the love, the kind words, the expressions that a daughter wants to hear from a father and a mother. She came away very satisfied."

"What about now?" I asked Mark. "Do you have a relationship with her parents?"

"Yes," he responded, "but we're not real close. It's interesting but Jennifer's mom just recently had a mastectomy, but nobody knew about it. She is a very private person. The only reason I even knew about it was that she called me the night before the surgery because she wanted me to let the kids know. She thought it might be devastating for Mike and Tonya to learn about it, so she wanted me to break it to them. I talked to her a while that night and again at the hospital right after the mastectomy. A week later we talked again but in all those conversations, there was no hint whatsoever of weakness or emotion. And, that's exactly how she took the news of Jennifer's terminal illness. She was and is a stoic, matter-of-fact lady who does not express any of her feelings."

"How is she doing now?" I asked.

"Well, the last time I talked to her she was doing fine," Mark said. "She came to visit us and she looked like her old self again. As far as I know, she's doing well. I haven't heard otherwise."

"Given Jennifer's situation, I wonder if she felt like her breast cancer was a death sentence," Rich said.

"I wondered that," Mark replied. "I didn't probe it with her. I didn't think it was my place to, but I certainly wondered that myself. It had to have crossed her mind, but I doubt she would ever express those thoughts to me."

"What about Tonya?" I asked. "How did her grandmother's mastectomy make her feel, especially after losing her mom to breast cancer?"

"Well, to be honest, I'm not real sure," Mark answered. "But before Jennifer died she talked with Tonya about the fact that Tonya was at risk for breast cancer. She explained to her the things she would have to do to protect herself. I've never spoken to Tonya personally about it. I never hear her dwell on it. I have a sense, however, that she's not overly concerned. Maybe that stems from the fact that as a young person you somehow feel immortal. You don't feel like anything bad is going to happen to you. I know that she realizes she is at risk. She is a very levelheaded young woman. I'm sure she will take all the necessary precautions."

"No one is useless in this world who lightens the burdens of it for another." - *Charles Dickens*

It continued to be a bright fall day. The sun was warm, yet not hot. The air felt clean and the breeze against our faces was refreshing. Sunbathers down the beach were gradually leaving.

"What about the kids, Mark," I said. "Did they express difficulty dealing with a future without their Mom in it?"

Mark paused for a couple minutes then began. "Tonya and I were pretty close and she would open up. Mainly she talked about missing out on all the things a mom would do with a daughter – going through the dating years, the wedding, the early stages of marriage, and the counsel that she would receive. Then there would be the grandchildren. It bothered Tonya a lot that her mom would not know her grandchildren. Those were the things that were preeminent in both Jennifer's and Tonya's mind. You know, a daughter needs her mother. A mother needs to be there for her daughter. Those were the main concerns, I think."

"Mike, though, is a pretty quiet guy. He didn't really share his feelings with me. All of his feelings and emotions were expressed with his mother. I remember coming home for lunch one time when Jennifer was thin and so ill. It was the most tender, intimate thing I'd ever witnessed in my life."

Mark paused, tried to talk but was overwhelmed by emotion and tears. The pitch of his voice rose as he struggled to describe the scene. "They had no idea that I was headed home. I didn't normally come home for lunch. I remember walking through the door and they were in the living room. Jennifer was in her pajamas and robe . . . . " Mark's tears turned to sobbing as he paused again. As he continued we worked hard to decipher his words.

"You remember our large wooden rocking chair. It was the chair that Jennifer used to rock and nurse her babies. Mike sat there holding his mom in that rocking chair like you would hold a little baby. He had his arm under her head and his other arm under her legs. He was just rocking and rocking and rocking her. She was lying with her head on his shoulder." Mark paused again, unable to control the sobbing and tears.

"Here's this tall, husky, tender young man who is so private with his emotions," he continued, "cradling and rocking his emaciated mom in the chair where she had once cradled and rocked him. It was overwhelming! It was a very intimate moment between a son and his mother. Their heads were together and they were communicating their love for each other. . . . . it was beautiful." Mark paused again. More tears. "I was so taken back by that, I actually backed out of the room. It was personal and compassionate. I didn't want to interrupt it. I quietly left the house so they wouldn't know I was there."

Sobbing continued, except now it was us sobbing right along with Mark. We knew Mike and his quiet nature and were deeply moved by the scene Mark had placed in our minds. What a wonderful, loving moment it must have been for Jennifer. What a tender memory it must be for Mike. Our conversation paused as we all composed ourselves.

"Let's walk down the beach a bit," Rich said, stretching as he got up from the picnic table.

"That sounds good to me," Mark replied.

We headed up the beach with the sun midway to the western horizon. A child's toy laid on the sand, half buried and overlooked by the chubby mom in the bikini who had just left in a gold minivan. Mark stooped down, picked up the toy, rubbed the sand from its creases and held it to himself like a security blanket. His large stature dramatized the action, yet as he walked and held his treasure, a small boy seemed to emerge from within. With childlike innocence and honesty he opened and exposed his heart.

"I don't know how other people handle it when a spouse is terminally ill. I know for me, it was a mixed bag. Here was this woman I had known since middle school. We sorta grew up together. I dated her in high school. We married at 19. I'd spent most of my life with her. When we got married we were still kids but there was a strong bond between us. I had an intense love for Jennifer. There was the part of me that grieved the pending loss of all that. It was a real and deep grief. And then, there was the other part of me. It was the part that knew her death was inevitable, and I looked towards the future. I thought about the possibilities of meeting and marrying someone else. In a sense, that's an adventure. It was exciting to think about those things. Yet at the same time when I thought about it or I dwelled on that, I felt guilty."

"It was like: how can I even be thinking about these things – my wife's dying! It was a tug of war. It was back and forth. It was an incredibly painful time. Fortunately the kids were at an age where I had no real concerns about them and what would happen to them. They were young adults. Had they been younger, it would have been totally different."

"It is so difficult living with someone who is terminally ill. On the one hand you have to get up and go to work every day. You know, life doesn't just stop because of the illness. You have bills to pay. You've got responsibilities. I had just started a new job and I wanted to do well. I wanted to excel. I'm competitive and I had ambitions. I wanted to make my mark in the world. At that time I was 42 years old. I was at the height of my career. Then, on the other hand, always in the back of my mind was my wife who was dying. When I went home I had to deal with that. For the first year of her illness it wasn't an inconvenience because Jennifer was pretty healthy and mobile. She was ambulatory and all that. But then she started getting progressively weaker. She couldn't go anywhere. She couldn't do anything. I'd come home and she'd be on the couch in her pajamas. She had this terrible itching of her skin, as you recall, then there would be bleeding. She wasted away. She started needing more physical care; not that I did a lot of physical care because Jennifer was a very strong-willed and private woman. There were only a few times that I actually would bath her and care for her in a physical sense like that. Tonya left college to come home and care for her at the last. All in all, it was very disheartening. To see her wasting away before my eyes was extremely depressing. Yet the next day, I had to go to work and people didn't want to hear about that. I was there to counsel. I was there to lift the hearts of the people."

"Whereas there were many victories in my home life, you know, small types of victories where I felt an answer to a prayer or some joy that was expressed even in the midst of heartache, the overwhelming sense of it was just very depressing."

"What were some of the things you did to cope?" I asked.

"I walked a lot. That was my number one coping mechanism. There was a time when I would walk for hours. That's how I escaped in a sense. Sometimes it bordered on obsession. I can remember very distinctly walking a few times for four or five hours. A couple of times I went out in the middle of winter in subzero temperatures. It was my way of escaping reality."

"Another coping mechanism was that I constructed a fantasy world. What I mean by that is a world of the future. I tried to envision what that would be. I dwelled on that quite a bit. It wasn't something I could share with Jennifer because that would be too hurtful. Jennifer and I basically our whole lives shared everything together. I don't think that we had any secrets at all up until we started parting ways – she started down one path and I started down another. There were things I couldn't share with her any more. You know, though, I probably could have. She was mature enough that she might have been able to handle some of it. But I didn't feel like I could and I didn't. I remember that on my long walks I created fantasies in my mind, none of which materialized. They were unrealistic. There was no basis in reality."

"What about the kids, Mark," Rich asked. "Do you think they did anything to escape? How did they cope?"

"I'm sorry that I don't know more," Mark slowly responded. "I guess our talking has been kind of revealing to me – how glaring my understanding is of what the kids were going through. Maybe I was too self-absorbed at the time. I don't know. I didn't understand what the kids were feeling. I don't know how they coped. It's not that we didn't try to approach the subject with the kids. But Mike, especially, was very, very, closed mouthed. I didn't always know what he was thinking or feeling. So, I don't know how they coped or what they did."

"I really regret that I lived in a fantasy world too much that last year. I regret that I wasn't fully there for Jennifer. I mean I was there physically. I was there when she needed me in every way. I was kind to her. I was gentle with her. I was supportive to her. We did things together. We had intimate times together. I was there in all those ways. Outwardly I was there. But what I regret as much as anything is that I wasn't fully focused on her and what she was going through. I couldn't be there for her like that, and I wished I could have. I wished my whole being would have been there supporting her but I was living in some fantasy world out there somewhere. As a result of that, I wasn't there and I regret that terribly. I regret it terribly."

Mark walked with his head down, still clutching the child's toy he found up the beach. He walked lightly and then kicked at the sand every few steps.

"What are some things you wish Jennifer would have done that she didn't do?" I asked. "Was there anything?"

Mark lifted his head, looked out across the water and paused long before he began.

"I wish Jennifer had left a larger legacy. By that I mean I wish I had more photos, more video tapes, audio tapes and letters. I wish I had her writings wherein she expressed her feelings and her thoughts. I miss that. My memory is not as

92

good as I wish it was, and things become hazy after a while. I would have liked for her to have written her thoughts down so that I could review them on occasion and go back and remember. Jennifer was a very wise person. She sized up people and situations very quickly. I'd like to hear some of her wisdom from time to time. I remember some of the wise things that she said. It would have been nice to impart some of those things to her children and grandchildren."

"Jennifer was such a vital part of my life. We spent 24 years of marriage and dated two or three years before that. We were together a vast part of my life. I miss not having her to kind of spark my memory. I miss the sense of history that she brought to our family. She was the repository of the history, of the stories of when the kids were little and growing. She was basically raising them while I was either in the Army or was away at school. I was trying to forge a career for myself and Jennifer was the one who raised the kids for the most part. She had all the stories. I don't have the stories. I miss that. That's what makes you a family."

"Jennifer was so funny. She had great stories that only she could tell. I've tried to tell some of them and I might be able to get a laugh, but when she'd tell them, she'd have people rolling on the floor. She had a unique way of telling funny stories."

Beginning to laugh, I responded, "I miss her stories, too. She did have a real gift. I love the closet story. You don't know how many times I've burst out laughing as I've envisioned her hiding when the parsonage committee dropped in."

"That was a funny story," Mark laughed. "She told it so well. She had lots of stupid little stories like that. Only Jennifer could get into such predicaments. I really miss all the remembrances. I can't always connect the dots. She was my storehouse of remembrances. I miss her so."

"In addition to leaving a larger legacy for us, there's maybe another thing I wish Jennifer had done differently. I know this is going to sound strange, but I wish that at times during her struggle with cancer she would have gotten angrier with me. You and I have talked during the past about how Jennifer handled anger. You said to me that she shared with you times that she was angry with different people or at situations. But she didn't share a lot of that with me. I didn't see Jennifer angry a lot. I can remember constantly feeling guilty about my failings of her during that time. I felt guilty also because of the fact that I was going to survive and have a life beyond and she wasn't. I felt guilty for thinking ahead to that time in my life: what I would do, the people I would date; perhaps the person I would marry and things like that. Maybe if she had been angry with me, I'd have felt less guilty."

"I've never told anybody this. While Jennifer and Mike were on their trip to visit Jennifer's parents, the house was pretty empty and quiet. There was a sense of relief for me during that time. It wasn't a sick house any more. At the time, I was working with a bunch of young college kids and, of course, Tonya still lived there. She was a part of that group. So, almost every night the college kids would come over and we'd laugh and play games. We played cards and stayed up till all hours of the night having a good time. There was a feeling of release for me. I began to think about my future and wonder if this was what it could be like. When Jennifer got back home something happened. I don't really recall what it was, but we had a falling out."

Laughingly I said, "Was it maybe because the house was a mess? I do seem to recall something like that." The three of us laughed as Rich gave Mark a shove towards the water.

"That could be," Mark laughed. "I don't remember what it was, but it was a very serious time and I remember I deliberately wanted to hurt Jennifer. I wanted to say something that was hurtful to her. I was going through a lot of turmoil and I remember telling her very distinctly that I didn't love her any more." Mark paused and began again. His voice was quivering and was much softer. " . . . . . And . . . . ah . . . . and I emphasized that several times to her. . . . . . and I remember she took it in perfect stride. She never reacted to it. She never got angry. She simply reminded me

94

that I did love her, that she knew that I loved her, no matter what I said or did, that would never change. That just ripped through my heart. How could I have been so foolish and cruel? Maybe if she had gotten angry with me I would have felt less guilty about that. As it is, I feel guilty to this day that I said those dumb words. It was so stupid."

"Why did you want to hurt her?" I asked. Mark repeated the question to himself and after a long pause he replied. "I was tired of the whole thing. It was a long drawn out nightmare, such a daily reminder. It was so painful. I was impatient. She was the source of all that pain, not her, but her illness. But it was hard to separate the two. I don't know exactly why I said it in that moment other than it was at the end of a period of time where I had felt a reprieve and life was good. But, Jennifer knew my heart and that's what counts. Even though I said those mean, ugly, terrible words which I wished I could have taken back, she knew my heart."

"If you concentrate on finding whatever is good in every situation, you will discover that your life will suddenly be filled with gratitude, a feeling that nurtures the soul."
- *Rabbi Harold Kushner*

A hundred thoughts swirled through my mind as we turned to walk back up the beach toward our cars. "What are some things you wish you could have read about in a book during the time of Jennifer's illness," I asked Mark.

"That's a good question. Primarily, I guess I would loved to have read about people who were going through what we were at the time," he responded. "I don't mean someone who made everything sugary sweet – you know – 'It all works out in the end. It was a wonderful, victorious walk. She went home to be with the Lord and she's in a resurrected body. Now everybody lives happily ever after.' You know what I'm talking about. I think what would have been most helpful was to have read about the real rawness of the truth of someone's experiences during a time like that. I have read all my life. I've read hundreds of books. The best books I have read are those that are real and don't gloss things over. I would have appreciated a book that described the real struggles people go through. Those are the types of things that would have helped – a balance between the positive and the harsh realities. Not that you don't come out on the high side. I mean that's the goal, of course. You want to get there. But it's not an unbroken path. It's strewn with lots of potholes and rocks. It's very painful. You're going to fail and be hurt and hurt others. And yet in all of that you hopefully achieve some measure of victory over those things."

"I think as far as Jennifer, she would have loved to have found a book that answered the "why" question. But, of course, who of us is wise enough to put that down on paper? There was no answer in scripture that we could find. There were no answers in any of the writings that we read. Why would God allow Jennifer, a good woman, a fine woman . . . . . why? There's no answer to that. That's what she would have wanted to find. I don't think that in the end that question was answered for her, although she had peace in spite of not knowing why. That's what faith is, is it not? Really, truly. To experience peace and a sense of acceptance even when you have all those unanswered questions. Reading about people who demonstrate a victory over adversity is the most uplifting type of reading. I love that kind. Jennifer loved it. She loved to read about people who were physically healed, of course, because she sought to number herself among those same people. But equally important was to read about people who simply overcame adversity and who were victorious in spite of the fact that there was no lasting healing – where there was no victory over whatever area they were struggling. It's not important to know all of the warts and blemishes, but to just know that they are there. It was not an unbroken track of faith that Jennifer and I experienced where we just soared. It was a very human drama and every human drama is filled with all kinds of heartache and pain."

"Mark, what are the things you think of on those days when you miss Jennifer?" Rich asked. "Well," he slowly began. "I will share with you some intimate moments if you would permit it. When I think of Jennifer now, I often think of the times that we made love. Jennifer and I married at 19 and we were both virgins at that time. We remained faithful our whole married lives. I never knew another woman except Jennifer, and I am quite confident that she never knew another man."

"When I think of her now, I think back to some of those wonderful moments. Interestingly enough the times that are most pronounced in my remembrances are the first time we made love and the last time we made love. There were other wonderful mountaintop experiences in between, but they were few and far between. There was the time she came up to Fort Dix to visit me while I was in the Army. We had no place to go to be alone except into a cornfield. We hadn't seen each other in six months and we made love in a cornfield. I remember the time right after she found out that she had breast cancer, before her mastectomy. We went to a deserted island and in broad daylight made love on the sand dunes. Those were wonderful moments. But, the most memorable for me are the first time, our wedding night, and the last time before she died. Both of those were very special, tender moments."

"I'd like to tell you a little something about the last time. We didn't have much of a sex life through that last year. A couple months before Jennifer died she had been suffering quite a bit, but she asked me specifically one night if I would make love to her. I said that I would, I mean I was delighted to. It was a very tender moment. There was not the passion of youth, the exuberance of youth, the physicality of youth and all of that, but there was tenderness. And, there was also a deliberate knowledge that this would probably be the last time we would spend intimate moments together as man and wife. I remember that so clearly."

"As I thought about that, I've thought about how our love changed over the years. When I first met Jennifer she was so young and beautiful. She had such a beautiful body. It was a perfect body, and I loved her in a physical sense. We shared a physical romantic kind of love. As we grew older she had the children and age came upon her, and her body wasn't quite as beautiful because of child bearing and putting on weight. I remember that I began to love her for the things that she did in our marriage. She was a wonderful mother, a fabulous homemaker, a skilled nurse, and a great friend. She was all those things. I loved her for the things that she did for the family and me. Then she reached the last stage of her life when she was no longer physically beautiful because the disease had ravaged her body and the mastectomy had scarred her. We used to laugh because she said I had the best of both worlds. I had a flat-chested

98

woman and I had a full-breasted woman. During the last stage of her life she no longer could do the things she used to do. She couldn't wait on the family and couldn't work as a nurse any more. She couldn't do any of the things I had grown to love and appreciate. I had to look deeper. I knew that I loved Jennifer for the person she was. I think this is the deepest kind of love. I loved her for her character, for her honor and for her faithfulness. I loved her for the strength that she brought to this trial in her life. I loved her for the nobility, the humility and all those wonderful, wonderful traits that came out during her suffering. They were always there as part of who she was, but they were made prominent during her illness."

"When I think of Jennifer it's often times in the context of loving her in all those different ways. I have a 24-year span when Jennifer was young, beautiful and had a gorgeous body, then in middle age when she was heavier set, then at the end when she was scarred and sick. I get to pick and choose which level of love to reflect on in each of the different times of our life together. Those are wonderful memories," he smiled.

It was good to have met Mark at the beach on the first anniversary of Jennifer's death. It was fitting to have shared our feelings and reunited in our love for her. The world we once knew had totally changed. Greater changes would assuredly take place and life would continue to evolve, but our love for Jennifer was unchanging. We did a group hug as we left the beach and headed back to our cars to continue further into our new phase of life.

Several years after our providential meeting with Mark, Rich and I planned a trip to visit him. Much had happened to all of us since that afternoon at the beach. Rich and I became grandparents and experienced the wonderful joys of our expanded family. Mark remarried and was living several hundred miles away. He told us that he had become reunited with Lisa, a girl he had known in school. "She was the first girl I ever kissed," he told us. "I hadn't seen her since high school."

As Mark approached us at the airport he carried himself erect and almost appeared younger than when we last saw him. His smile was large as he greeted us. "You guys look great! You haven't changed a bit," he laughed.

"Yeah," Rich mocked, "and your nose is going to grow if you keep telling those lies!" We gathered our luggage from the carousel and headed out of the airport.

"So tell us about Lisa," Rich said as we got in the car. "What's she like?"

"Oh, she's really great," Mark responded. "You will like her. She's a remarkable woman for many reasons, but in this sense in particular. She has never felt threatened by my memories of Jennifer. I remember very early on in our relationship that she encouraged me to talk about Jennifer. She wanted to hear about her. She wanted to hear about my love for Jennifer and our love for each other. She wanted to know the things we shared together. She's said, and repeated it often, that the fact that I loved Jennifer so much gives her a sense of security in knowing that if I'm capable of loving Jennifer like that, then I'm capable of loving her like that as well. I have a picture of Jennifer on my dresser and I have a picture of Lisa on my dresser. Lisa's never been threatened by that. I don't have a lot of other pictures of Jennifer. I do have a lot of things of Jennifer's, but that's primarily because I love those things as well. I'll never get rid of the stained glass window she made. That's a permanent possession. I'll give it to Tonya some day, but Lisa doesn't seem to be threatened by any of it. I'm very fortunate."

"Are you happy?" I asked, hoping for an affirmative answer. "I am," he replied, "but I still feel the loss of family the kids and I had. I miss Jennifer's ability to make us a family. She was the glue that held us all together. When she died we were fragmented terribly. Part of it was the stage of life the kids were in. Tonya went back to college and Mike was out on his own building a business. Then all of a sudden I was the only parent to make a home, if and when they returned for the holidays. I mean there was

100

nothing there. And even to this day we don't have a central focus. Lisa tries, but she doesn't share the traditions. She doesn't share the memories. She doesn't share the history that the kids and I have. Tonya has tried to step into that role. During the holidays, especially Thanksgiving or Christmas, Tonya has tried to do things like her mom. She likes to serve the same dishes that her mother served. She enjoys decorating the tree and the house and organizing the holidays the way in which her mom did. She tries to do all those things that we had come to appreciate and love so. I really miss the sense of family Jennifer brought to us."

"I think the kids were devastated, there's no doubt about that in my mind. And, our sense of family was the greatest loss that we experienced. It didn't help that so many miles separated us. Even to this day that's the thing that the kids remark about. Six months ago Tonya said she wanted to quit working. One of the reasons was that she wanted to spend more time creating a family life for us. We have a family business and we see each other every day. We work closely with each other. But what we don't do is sit down and eat together. We don't spend weekends doing fun things with each other. Holidays are somewhat disjointed now because Lisa has her family that she likes to spend some holidays with, and rightfully so. Sometimes that pulls us away on Thanksgiving or Christmas and it's not the same. If I'm not there, it changes the equation for the kids. So what Tonya wants to do is have supper at least once a week and cook some of the old recipes. She wants to make sure that holidays are special family occasions. She wants to plan family outings, maybe something as simple as going to a movie and eating out together."

"Tonya's a wonderful gal," I responded. "What a great tribute to her mom for her to want to emulate and pick up the slack. You must be very proud of her. Tell me, how long did it take before you really felt like life was good again?"

"Hummmmm," Mark responded. "I'm just now experiencing all that I believe. It took a career change. It took a new marriage. It took starting a family business. It took giving up unrealistic dreams. It's taken a long time and I'm just now starting to feel good about my life again. As I've thought about it, it truly has been a deliberate rebuilding of my life. One of the fascinating things about surviving the death of a spouse and having children at the age where they were starting life on their own is that my life was like a clean slate. It really was. In the past I had started down a certain career pathway and I needed to continue that because I had obligations. I had responsibilities. I had bills to pay. I had to provide for my family. After doing something for 20 years it's pretty hard to give that up and go follow a dream."

"But when Jennifer died, it was like I had a fresh start. I could do anything I wanted to do. I could go anywhere that I wanted to go. I had no one to be responsible to except for myself and occasionally to the kids. So, there was a deliberate rebuilding. I began to make decisions based on what I wanted to do for the rest of my life. That's a wonderful gift to receive. It's also a heavy weight. It's starting all over again in a sense. I felt like I had achieved some success and some confidence in my previous life and my previous career. Starting all over again was difficult. I think there were a few false starts along the way. But I think that now I have chosen wisely. I have chosen a field that I am vastly interested in. I love the challenges of running a business, of having a family business. I feel like my life is, for the first time since before Jennifer got sick, fairly stable. We are putting down roots into a community. Always before as a pastor I didn't get deeply involved in the community other than our church because I knew I'd only live there a few years. But now, I see this community as the place where I will live and die. I don't have any grand allusions that I'm going to move someplace else or find something more exciting to do. This is my life and I'm starting to enjoy it, letting loose of some of the past, accepting the present and trying not to live into the future."

CHAPTER 14   AN EPILOGUE

"Blessed is the influence of one true, loving human soul on another." - George Eliot

A hotel was the setting for the conference. As I entered the large room during a break I noticed Mickey sitting at a table near the center of the room. She smiled wide as our eyes met and she beckoned me to her table. Her dark hair accented her large brown eyes. Her cream linen dress showed off her trim figure. By far she was the prettiest woman at the conference. Her outer beauty though was far surpassed by her inner beauty. She was wise beyond her years. Her life experiences had been difficult but she maintained a tender spirit. We hugged as we greeted each other and I took the chair next to hers.

"It's so good to see you, Mickey," I said. "I didn't know you would be here."

"It's good to see you, too," she returned. Handing her camera to a friend, Mickey said, "Please take our picture." I pulled my chair closer to Mickey's and put my arm around her shoulder. I thought of Jennifer as we smiled at the lens and the camera clicked.

Years earlier Mickey and I had breast surgery about the same time. In comparing notes about our surgeries, I had told Mickey that I woke up during my surgery and had started talking to the doctor. He told me that things were looking pretty good.

"I woke up during my surgery, too," Mickey had told me. "But I woke up to the doctor saying 'Oh, no! How old is she?' Just like you, I knew the outcome before the surgery was even over, except mine wasn't as good as yours."

Mickey had undergone chemo following her surgery and other treatments as the cancer spread. Her eyes were bright and her smile continuous as we talked together during the conference break. We discussed our kids and her health.

"How are you doing, Mickey?" I asked.

With calmness in her voice she said, "I've been pretty sick. The cancer has continued to spread and the prognosis is not good. It's terminal. If I had known what I know now," Mickey said slowly, "I wouldn't have had my stomach removed. It was so difficult, painful and ultimately disappointing. It didn't stop the cancer and I can't do it any more. I'm done with treatment and surgery," she resolutely said. "No more."

"I'm sorry, Mickey, that you've been through so much," I said. "I'm really sorry."

"I know you are," she returned with tears in her eyes. "But do you know what?" Mickey interjected quickly with excitement. "I met your friend, Jennifer, at a wedding a couple months before she died. I had heard about her, of course, from you and from some other mutual friends. It was so good to meet her and spend some time talking. She was an amazing lady."

"That she was," I agreed. "You know," Mickey continued, "she did it all so well. She handled her illness with such grace and confidence that everybody who heard about her was impressed. I was in awe of her strength. We had such a good talk. I want to do it just like her. I want to demonstrate and live out my faith with the same zeal she did. Her faith extended beyond expecting to be healed. She trusted God to work out His best plan for her and her family in spite of not being healed."

"She did, Mickey. She really did," I said, "and it's impressive that you courageously are following her example."

Mickey did do it well. She learned from Jennifer, then became a model for others to follow. Jennifer would be pleased to know how she impacted Mickey. She would be so glad to realize that her lonely walk made Mickey's difficult walk easier.

Mickey and Jennifer are together now. They're probably telling each other funny stories about the predicaments they got themselves into here on earth. Maybe they're comparing notes about the things that bugged them during their illnesses. Perhaps they're writing the rest of Jennifer's book, remembering to be generous in the last chapter with their forgiveness of us, their friends and family, who didn't always know how to effectively help them during their walk through terminal illness. I'm proud to have been their friend. I'm grateful for the lessons they taught me. May their lessons live on to encourage others on their lonely walks.

They demonstrated so fully that life is about engaging ourselves in the present in spite of what the future might promise. It's about living with hope when things appear hopeless. It's about looking for and finding beauty in the midst of adversity. It's about dreaming your dreams and discovering new courage. It's about finding a smile when it'd be easier to cry. It's about being thankful to be able to wash dishes. It's about maintaining dignity in spite of indignities. It's about claiming purpose and meaning in each moment. It's about celebrating life every day. It's about trusting God to work out His best plan.

Do you have thoughts on discovering hope and courage during difficult days? What are your suggestions for supporting others during challenging times?

I'd be interested in hearing from you. Please e-mail your comments and ideas to Anna Lynn at:

annalynn16354@yahoo.com

Examples shared by others:

When supporting our family during a time of difficulty, people brought food to the house in disposable dishes. This eliminated the burden for me having to remember what dishes belonged to whom and then having to return them.   – Jacob

During chemotherapy treatment I was unable to properly clean my house. The ladies of my church knew that if they came to clean, it would have a dual impact on me. First of all, I would be embarrassed to have them see my dirty house. Second, I would feel an obligation to leave my bed to talk with them. They knew I needed my rest and didn't want me to be embarrassed by the condition of my house, so they did a very kind and creative thing that I greatly appreciated. They hired a professional cleaner to clean my house for me. They were assured the job would be done well and I did not feel obligated to socialize while she was cleaning. It was a wonderful gift.   - Madison

During a period of time when I was very sick, my friends took turns baking cookies for my kids. I kept the cookies next to my bed and I was able to give my children a treat, even though I was physically unable to bake the cookies myself. It allowed me the privilege of expressing love and comfort to my children in this way during a season that was difficult for them, as well as for me. - Delaney

Do say, "I'm sorry." Don't say, "It's okay." When my mother died suddenly, a nurse in the hospital emergency room extended her arms to comfort me as she said, "It's okay." I pulled away from her as her words repelled me. I wanted to snap at her, "It's not okay! She's my mother! She just died. IT'S NOT OKAY!" I was devastated by my mother's death. Had the nurse simply said, "I'm sorry," I could have found comfort in her words.   - Keeley

My husband was diagnosed with terminal lung cancer. He was a real people person. He enjoyed being with all his friends, but since his illness, they were reluctant to just drop in to visit because he was so sick. During a good week for him I had an open house one Saturday afternoon. I asked people to stop in for a few minutes and visit us. The kids helped me make cookies, punch and coffee. Our friends came, assured that their visit was not inconvenient for us, but welcome. It was a wonderful day of laughter and warmth. He loved it. - Bev

My wife had regularly been going to help her terminally ill friend. One day as she visited, her friend said, "Becky, I really appreciate you coming, but I'm not up to talking today." Becky told her that was okay, and she simply sat at the foot of her friend's bed and rubbed her feet to make her more comfortable. - Brad

The best advice I'd give a caregiver is to take care of you. It's very, very important to get proper sleep and rest. Sometimes you also need to take a break. I felt guilty if I took time for myself when I was caring for my wife. I learned, though, that you won't be able to do as much for others if you don't take care of yourself. You can't be afraid to ask for help. I was a retired Chief Master Sergeant in the Air Force when my wife got sick. I was used to handling problems, but her illness was something I couldn't fix. I focused on what needed to be done and didn't know I wasn't handling it well. After she died, I had two major attacks on my body. I'll never forget looking into the frightened face of my twelve-year-old daughter. She had just lost her mom and now EMTs were carrying me out of the house on a stretcher. The doctor said it was stress related. Stress can do weird things to your body and it pulls on you when you don't realize it. It's paramount to get the right amount of sleep and take breaks. You have to protect your body so you will be able to do the important things.   – Keith

"Each dawn holds a new hope for a new plan, making the start of each day the start of a new life." *- Gina Blair*

What is your story?

E-mail to Anna Lynn at <u>annalynn16354@yahoo.com</u>